MCQs for the MRCP Part 1

Clinical chemistry, haematology and infectious disease

Commissioning Editor: Laurence Hunter
Project Editor: Sarah Keer-Keer
Project Controller: Nancy Arnott
Designer: Erik Bigland

MCQs for the MRCP Part 1

Clinical chemistry, haematology and infectious disease

David Galvani
MD MRCP MRCPath
Consultant Haematologist, Wirral Hospital NHS Trust

Duncan Neithercut
MD MRCP FRCPath
Consultant Clinical Chemist, Department of Chemical Pathology
Wirral Hospital NHS Trust

Nick Beeching
MA FRCP FRACP DCH DTM&H
Consultant Physician, Infectious Disease Unit
University Hospital Aintree, Liverpool
& Senior Lecturer in Infectious Diseases
Liverpool School of Tropical Medicine, University of Liverpool

Fred Nye
MD FRCP
Consultant Physician, Infectious Disease Unit
University Hospital Aintree, Liverpool
& Director of Studies – Infectious Diseases, University of Liverpool

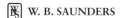 W. B. SAUNDERS

Edinburgh • London • New York • Philadelphia • Sydney • Toronto 1999

W.B. SAUNDERS
An imprint of Harcourt Brace and Company Limited

© Harcourt Brace & Company Limited 1999

🅡 is a registered trade mark of Harcourt Brace and Company Limited

The right of D. Galvani, W. Neithercut, N. Beeching and F. Nye to be identified as
authors of this work has been asserted by them in accordance with the Copyright,
Designs and Patents Act 1988.

First published 1999

ISBN 07020 2306X

British Library Cataloguing in Publication Data
A catalogue record for this book is available from the British Library.

Library of Congress Cataloging in Publication Data
A catalog record for this book is available from the Library of Congress.

Medical knowledge is constantly changing. As new information becomes available,
changes in treatment, procedures, equipment and the use of drugs become
necessary. The authors/editors/contributors and the publishers have, as far as it is
possible, taken care to ensure that the information given in this text is accurate and
up to date. However, readers are strongly advised to confirm that the information,
especially with regard to drug usage, complies with current legislation and standards
of practice.

The
publisher's
policy is to use
**paper manufactured
from sustainable forests**

Printed in China
EPC/01

Contents

Preface

Clinical chemistry, haematology and infectious disease are three areas in which students often have limited clinical experience. Questions in these areas often become 'deciders' in the MRCP Part 1 exam: separating those who pass from those who fail. Studying using this book will help candidates for the exam to become more proficient in these areas of particular difficulty.

The MCQs in this book have been regularly used on MRCP Part 1 candidates, and have ben revised and honed to suit their needs. The quesitons covern many exam 'chestnuts', but also include questions on recent developments and advances in clinical chemistry, haematology and infectious disease. Each question is answered in full, allowing testing and learning to occur simultaneously.

D.W. Galvani
1999

Acknowledgements

The authors would like to thank Dr Henry Mwandumba and Dr George Wyatt for their comments on the infectious disease section of this book.

Clinical chemistry

QUESTIONS

1. Consider the following statements concerning the interpretation of routine biochemical tests:
   a. Prolactin concentrations in serum may be used to determine whether apparent grand mal seizures are true or faked
   b. Thyroglobulin is not useful as a tumour marker to follow the progression of thyroid carcinoma
   c. Oxygen enhances the toxicity of paraquat and ingestion of only 2–3 g of paraquat substance can be fatal if untreated
   d. Rheumatoid factor is an IgG which, if present in a serum sample, is always diagnostic of rheumatoid arthritis
   e. The half-life of carboxyhaemoglobin in a patient breathing 21% oxygen is 4 h but this is reduced to 40 min on 100% oxygen

2. Which of the following conditions might produce an abnormal response during the short dexamethasone test?
   a. Endogenous depression
   b. Alcoholism
   c. Dementia
   d. Anorexia
   e. Obesity

3. To activate vitamin D, cholecalciferol undergoes two hydroxylation steps: 25-hydroxylation by the liver and 1α-hydroxylation in the kidney. Besides PTH, a number of other hormones can stimulate the renal 1α-hydroxylation. Which of the hormones below can stimulate 1α-hydroxylation?
   a. Growth hormone
   b. Cortisol
   c. Oestradiol
   d. Prolactin
   e. Thyroxine

4. Consider the following statements concerning the effects of alcohol on metabolism.

   a. Carbon tetrachloride is more hepatoxic in alcoholics because of reduced metabolism of the substance due to a reduction in the activity of the hepatic microsomal oxidase systems

   b. Alcohol and acetaldehyde can directly inhibit oxidative phosphorylation and thereby damage mitochondria

   c. Alcohol dehydrogenase is a mitochondrial enzyme

   d. The hypogonadism which may result from alcohol consumption is not due to decreased testosterone synthesis

   e. Alcohol produces an increase in the hepatic cytosol NAD: NADH ratio which can result in lactic acidosis

5. In the syndrome of inappropriate antidiuresis:

   a. Plasma AVP (arginine vasopressin, ADH) levels are always raised

   b. Plasma AVP levels are suppressed

   c. There is end-organ insensitivity to AVP release

   d. There is loss of the hypothalamic control of AVP release

   e. There is no single pattern of abnormality of AVP concentrations in plasma in this syndrome

6. Match the vitamin with the appropriate associated clinical condition:

   a. Thiamine (B1)

   b. Vitamin C

   c. Nicotinic acid (niacin)

   d. Excess of vitamin A

   e. Folic acid

   1. A combination of angular stomatitis, diarrhoea, raw beef tongue, erythema, mental changes

   2. Neural tube defects

   3. Wernicke's encephalopathy

   4. Liver damage

   5. Scurvy

7. Match the metal with the appropriate associated clinical conditions:

   a. Selenium
   b. Cadmium
   c. Mercury
   d. Aluminium
   e. Lead

   1. Dialysis encephalopathy
   2. Blue line on the gums
   3. Monitored by urinary β_2-microglobulin measurement
   4. Muscle tremor, behavioural disturbance, sweating and salivation
   5. GI symptoms and a garlic-like odour in the breath, along with dry brittle hair

8. Match the type of porphyria with the correct metabolic abnormality:

   a. Porphyria cutanea tarda
   b. Erythropoietic protoporphyria
   c. Acute intermittent porphyria
   d. Variegate porphyria
   e. Lead poisoning

   1. Marked photosensitivity with an oedematous reaction
   2. Increased urinary 5-aminolaevulinate (ALA) and erythrocyte zinc protoporphyrin
   3. Deficiency of protoporphyrinogen oxidase
   4. Increased hepatic iron stores
   5. Increased urine excretion of porphobilinogen

9. Match the analytes with the appropriate clinical condition:

   a. Increased in alcoholic liver disease
   b. Increased in the acute-phase reaction
   c. Suppressed levels in a young woman may indicate pregnancy
   d. Of use in Down's syndrome screening
   e. Used in the management of germ cell malignancy

   1. Free β-HCG
   2. α-fetoprotein
   3. Caeruloplasmin
   4. Carbohydrate-deficient transferrin
   5. FSH and LH

10. Match the clinical condition associated with jaundice with the correct biochemical explanation:

    a. Dubin–Johnson syndrome
    b. Gilbert's syndrome
    c. Haemolytic anaemia
    d. Surgical obstructive jaundice
    e. Crigler–Najjar syndrome

    1. Mild unconjugated hyperbilirubinaemia and normal or decreased urinary urobilinogen
    2. Conjugated hyperbilirubinaemia with normal or decreased urobilinogen in the urine
    3. Marked unconjugated hyperbilirubinaemia with absence of urinary urobilinogen
    4. Mild unconjugated hyperbilirubinaemia with increased urinary urobilinogen
    5. Predominantly conjugated hyperbilirubinaemia with decreased urinary urobilinogen

11. In assessing the glomerular filtration rate, measurement of creatinine clearance is often used. Consider the following statements:

    a. The accuracy of creatinine clearance improves as renal function deteriorates due to loss of tubular function and thereby the capacity of the kidney to secrete creatinine
    b. Serial measurement of serum creatinine concentration may be as good a method of assessing deterioration in renal function as measuring creatinine clearance

c. The measurement of creatinine clearance is unaffected by dietary protein or exercise

d. A 24-h urine creatinine excretion of less than 6 mmol/24 h probably indicates an incomplete 24-h collection in men

e. A normal amylase creatinine clearance ratio occurs in macroamylasaemia

---

12. Regarding testing for cystic fibrosis:

a. Normal adults may have sweat sodium values greater than the upper limit of normal for children

b. A firm diagnosis of cystic fibrosis can be made solely on the basis of the measurement of sweat sodium using the pilocarpine iontophoresis technique of Gibson and Cooke

c. The gene for cystic fibrosis is autosomal recessive

d. Immunoreactive trypsin in blood spots may be used to screen for cystic fibrosis

e. In cystic fibrosis, there is a defect in the chloride ion transport across cell membranes

---

13. Consider the following statements concerning phaeochromocytoma:

a. Phaeochromocytoma is present in approximately 0.5% of hypertensive patients and 10% of cases may be familial

b. Phaeochromocytoma may occur in association with other endocrine neoplasms in MEN type 1

c. Bilateral phaeochromocytoma occurs more commonly in patients with familial phaeochromocytoma but overall approximately 10% of cases are familial

d. Postural hypotension may occur in patients with phaeochromocytoma and, if familial, may be helpful in making the clinical diagnosis

e. Patients should not eat bananas during urine collection for NMA analysis

14. What happens to serum hormone concentrations in pregnancy?

   a. The mean serum concentration of 17-hydroxyprogesterone rises three-fold by 40 weeks

   b. The mean serum testosterone concentration increases slightly during pregnancy

   c. The free androgen index rises during pregnancy, matching the change in testosterone concentration

   d. By the end of the pregnancy mean serum prolactin concentrations are as high as 3000 IU/l

   e. Placental DHEAS is the major source of oestrogens which rise during pregnancy although DHEAS concentrations are found to fall during the first half of pregnancy

15. Pancreatic exocrine and endocrine dysfunction may be monitored by a variety of tests:

   a. The 6-min insulin C-peptide response to 1 mg of IV glucagon may be used as a test of insulin reserve

   b. Macroamylasaemia when renal function is not impaired indicates chronic pancreatitis

   c. Pancreatic pseudocysts may be associated with a pleural fluid amylase concentration greater than that found in serum

   d. Serum lipase activity is a more sensitive marker of acute pancreatitis than amylase activity

   e. The glucagon test has been used for the diagnosis of insulinoma

16. A TSH concentration suppressed below the reference range does *not* occur in which of the following conditions?

   a. Graves' disease

   b. Viral thyroiditis

   c. Old age

   d. Hypopituitarism

   e. Sick euthyroid syndrome

17. Concerning uric acid metabolism:

   a. Individuals with gout always have a raised serum uric acid concentration

b. Uric acid is one of the principal antioxidants present in plasma
c. Serum uric acid levels are reduced in the Lesch–Nyhan syndrome
d. Uric acid crystals are deposited only in joints in patients with gout
e. Measurement of urine uric acid excretion may be used to decide on the most appropriate treatment for hyperuricaemia

18. Hyponatraemia is most commonly caused by:

a. Diuretic treatment
b. Excessive drinking of water
c. Cortisol deficiency
d. Failure to excrete water and sodium
e. Marked hyperlipidaemia

19. Polycystic ovarian syndrome may be associated with:

a. A reduced LH:FSH ratio
b. A raised testosterone concentration
c. A raised LH:FSH ratio
d. Hirsutism
e. Alopecia

20. Concerning α_1-antitrypsin deficiency:

a. α_1-antitrypsin deficiency always results in emphysema
b. The association of α_1-antitrypsin deficiency with other factors such as air pollution causes emphysema
c. α_1-antitrypsin is a protease inhibitor
d. α_1-antitrypsin deficiency may cause cystic liver disease in children
e. Family screening for α_1-antitrypsin deficiency is important

21. Match the correct interpretation of the arterial blood gas results:

	pH	H⁺	pCO_2		pO_2	
			kPa	mmHg	kPa	mmHg
a.	7.31	49	6.7	48	7.3	54
b.	7.58	27	3.2	24	13.4	104
c.	7.31	49	1.3	11	15.0	112
d.	7.58	27	6.8	49	16.3	122
e.	7.30	50	6.7	47	4.5	34

1. Metabolic alkalosis
2. Venous blood
3. Metabolic acidosis
4. Respiratory alkalosis
5. Respiratory acidosis

22. Match the pattern of LFTs with the most likely diagnosis:

	Alb (36–52)	Bil (5–21)	AST (<40)	ALT (<40)	GGT (11–50)	ALP (30–125)
a.	50	32	20	24	47	112
b.	42	69	524	689	976	200
c.	38	18	72	94	724	621
d.	24	74	18	22	46	127
e.	32	96	44	32	252	324

1. Primary biliary cirrhosis
2. Gilbert's syndrome
3. Viral hepatitis
4. End-stage cirrhosis
5. Hepatic metastases

23. Match the thyroid function test results with the information given:

	T4	TSH	Age (years)
a.	144	17.2	23
b.	44	4.3	54
c.	145	3.2	65
d.	116	<0.05	82
e.	189	0.4	26

1. Euthyroid, asymptomatic
2. Increased thyroxine-binding globulin
3. Poor compliance with treatment
4. Sick euthyroid
5. Adequate replacement

24. Hypocalcaemia without hyperphosphataemia may occur as a result of the following conditions:

   a. Frusemide treatment
   b. Transfusion of citrated blood
   c. Medullary carcinoma of the thyroid
   d. Pseudohypoparathyroidism
   e. Magnesium deficiency

25. Serum lactate dehydrogenase activity is *not* raised in which of the following conditions?

   a. Congestive cardiac failure
   b. Hypothyroidism
   c. Pernicious anaemia
   d. Diabetes mellitus
   e. Legionnaire's disease

26. Which of the following conditions are *not* associated with Addison's disease?

   a. Hypothyroidism
   b. Vitiligo
   c. Primary ovarian failure
   d. Pernicious anaemia
   e. Hyperparathyroidism

27. Considering the results of a glucose tolerance test:

    a. A 1-h glucose value of 13.0 mmol/l or more indicates diabetes mellitus

    b. The fasting glucose value must be within the reference range for a healthy population

    c. The exact timing of the 2-h blood sample is critical for the correct interpretation of the test

    d. A glucose tolerance test can be used to diagnose reactive hypoglycaemia

    e. Measurement of glycosylated haemoglobin is a recognized alternative

28. Hyponatraemia due to salt depletion occurs with:

    a. Multiple myeloma

    b. Treatment with DDAVP

    c. Treatment with potassium-sparing diuretics

    d. A low-salt diet for hypertension

    e. Treatment with carbamazepine

29. Which of the following conditions can be associated with hypercalcaemia?

    a. Addison's disease

    b. Thiazide diuretic administration

    c. Idiopathic hypercalciuria

    d. Hypophosphatasia

    e. Paget's disease

30. Hypokalaemia may be caused by which of the following conditions?

    a. Theophylline overdose

    b. Hypercalcaemia

    c. Treatment of cardiac failure with an ACE inhibitor

    d. Cushing's syndrome

    e. Addison's disease

31. Some diseases or their treatment may interfere with the measurement of tests used for the monitoring of other conditions. Pair the disease with the test it may interfere with:

a. Thyrotoxicosis
b. Diabetic ketoacidosis
c. Temporal arteritis
d. Rheumatoid arthritis
e. Liver failure

1. Digoxin
2. Cortisol
3. Potassium
4. Creatinine
5. Fructosamine

32. Which of the following biochemical results are *not* known to occur in patients with Addison's disease?

a. Raised serum urea concentration
b. Raised serum calcium concentration
c. A normal serum potassium concentration
d. A normal serum sodium concentration
e. A suppressed plasma ACTH concentration

33. Which of the following biochemical abnormalities do *not* occur as a result of hypothyroidism?

a. Raised serum creatinine kinase concentration
b. Raised serum lactate dehydrogenase concentration
c. Hyponatraemia
d. Hypertriglyceridaemia
e. Hypocalcaemia

34. Which of the following conditions may cause ketoacidosis?

a. Renal tubular acidosis
b. Starvation
c. Alcoholic intoxication
d. Salicylate poisoning
e. Myophosphorylase deficiency

35. Match each condition with one appropriate associated biochemical abnormality:

a. Hypomagnesaemia
b. Hypocalcaemia
c. Hypokalaemia
d. Hypophosphataemia
e. Hyponatraemia

1. Chronic constipation
2. Diabetes mellitus
3. Respiratory depression
4. Stellate cataracts
5. Hypoparathyroidism

36. In a young adult female who develops hirsutism, which would be of *least* help in making a diagnosis?

a. 17α-OH progesterone
b. Serum cortisol
c. Sex hormone-binding globulin concentration
d. LH:FSH ratio in serum
e. Testosterone concentration

37. Which of the following statements concerning prostate-specific antigen (PSA) levels is true?

a. Detectable serum levels are never found in women
b. Digital rectal examination results in significantly raised levels
c. PSA is ideal for screening for prostate cancer
d. Urinary retention causes raised PSA levels
e. PSA levels are useful for screening for prostatic carcinoma because they do not change once individuals are fully adult

38. Which of the following commonly analysed serum constituents do *not* show a consistent temporal variation in concentration?

a. Serum cortisol concentration
b. Serum zinc concentration
c. Serum TSH concentration
d. Serum cholesterol concentration
e. Serum bilirubin concentration

39. Consider the following statements concerning dyslipidaemia:

   a. The mean total cholesterol concentration in patients with premature coronary artery disease is greater than 7.4 mmol/l

   b. Total cholesterol concentrations in serum are higher in summer than winter

   c. The optimal time for the measurement of total cholesterol concentration following myocardial infarction is 3 months after discharge from hospital

   d. Raised triglyceride concentrations alone do not indicate an increased risk of ischaemic heart disease

   e. Significant individual variation in fasting or non-fasting serum cholesterol concentrations means that for any one patient the cholesterol concentration should optimally be measured on up to four occasions before drug treatment is commenced

40. The single biochemical test accepted as the best available single indicator of thyroid function is:

   a. Total serum thyroxine concentration

   b. TSH measured by a sensitive assay

   c. A TRH test

   d. Free T3 measurement

   e. Free T4 measurement

41. Consider the following statements concerning hyperprolactinaemia:

   a. Raised serum prolactin levels may be found in the postpartum period

   b. Serum prolactin levels greater than 1000 IU/l always indicate a prolactinoma

   c. Galactorrhoea is always associated with a raised serum prolactin level

   d. Serum prolactin levels may fall on resting

   e. Falsely raised levels may be found due to big prolactin

42. Raised serum enzyme and protein levels may be due to specific diseases:

    a. A raised CKMB percentage greater than 20% excludes a macro-CK rather than a myocardial infarction

    b. Cholinesterase activity in serum is raised in liver disease

    c. Increased CK MM$_3$ isoform concentration is one of the earliest changes indicative of myocardial infarction

    d. Myoglobin measurement in serum is of use in the diagnosis of myocardial infarction although most myoglobin is found in the skeletal muscle

    e. A raised transferrin concentration occurs in haemochromatosis

43. Are the following statements true or false?

    a. The glomerular filtration rate of patients with diabetes mellitus can be raised early on in the disease

    b. The loss of small amounts of albumin in urine (microalbuminuria) in diabetics is a marker for the microvascular complications of diabetes mellitus

    c. Diabetic patients with nephrotic syndrome might complain of frothy urine

    d. A significant deterioration in renal function in diabetics might occur without either the serum urea or creatinine concentrations rising out of the reference ranges

    e. Diabetic microalbuminuria can be treated with angiotensin-converting enzyme inhibitors

44. Consider the following statements concerning serum growth hormone concentrations:

    a. In adults growth hormone levels decline with age

    b. A raised growth hormone level in an adult is diagnostic of acromegaly

    c. During the insulin tolerance test in normal subjects, the insulin-induced hypoglycaemia suppresses growth hormone levels; while during the glucose tolerance test, hyperglycaemia causes growth hormone levels to rise

    d. In children, growth hormone deficiency may be diagnosed by measuring growth hormone levels before and after 15 min of vigorous exercise

    e. In adults growth hormone levels are constant throughout the day

45. Which of the following have been demonstrated to be risk factors for the development of IHD?

   a. Raised Lp(a) concentrations
   b. Raised triglyceride concentrations
   c. Low fibrinogen concentrations
   d. Reduced vitamin C and vitamin E concentrations
   e. LDL subclass patterns

46. Match the appropriate condition with the appropriate laboratory results.

   a. Pseudohypoparathyroidism
   b. Tertiary hyperparathyriodism
   c. Paget's disease
   d. Osteomalacia
   e. Brown tumour

	PTH	ALP	Ca²⁺	Alb	Phosphate
1.	↑	↑	↑	N	↓
2.	N	↑	N	N	N
3.	↑	↑	N	N	↓
4.	↑	↑	↑	↓	↑
5.	↑	N	↓	N	↑

47. Consider the following statements:

   a. The specificity of a test is the percent positivity of the test in the presence of the disease it detects
   b. The sensitivity of a test is the percent negativity of the test in the absence of the disease it detects
   c. The prevalence of a disease is defined as the number of subjects with the disease in a year within the total population with the disease
   d. The incidence of a disease is the number of new cases per year per 100 000 population
   e. The receiver operator characteristic curve demonstrates the true sensitivity and specificity of a test depending on the prevalence of the condition in the population studied

---

48. Consider the following statements concerning nutrition:

    a. If hypoalbuminaemia is used to determine nutritional status then 50% or more of hospital patients in surgical wards are undernourished

    b. During total parenteral nutrition hyperglycaemia is less likely to occur as a complication if the initial blood glucose value is less than 10 mmol/l

    c. Patients in hospital following major surgical procedures have an increased total calorie requirement due to the catabolic response to the surgical insult (compared with their calorie requirement prior to surgery)

    d. Trace metal and essential fatty acid supplements should always be given to all patients requiring parenteral nutrition

    e. A glutamine supplement during parenteral feeding helps maintain bowel function

---

49. Consider the statements about tumour markers:

    a. Serum CA 125 levels may also be raised in patients with ascites

    b. Marginally raised CA 125 levels may be found in patients with endometriosis

    c. CA 153 may be raised in patients with breast carcinoma

    d. CA 153 is not raised in patients with chronic liver disease, tuberculosis or SLE

    e. Raised α-FP levels in patients with liver enzyme abnormalities indicate hepatoma

---

50. Consider the following statements:

    a. Serum troponin T levels are only raised following myocardial infarction

    b. Serial measurement of troponin T is needed for the confirmation of myocardial infarction

    c. A normal troponin T value on admission excludes myocardial infarction

    d. Mildly raised troponin T levels in patients with angina indicate a poorer prognosis

    e. Troponin T levels may remain raised for up to 2 weeks following myocardial infarction

1. a.**T** b.**F** c.**T** d.**F** e.**T**

True grand mal seizures may cause many biochemical abnormalities including lactic acidosis, hypoxia and raised stress hormone concentrations including raised serum prolactin concentrations. This is not the case following faked seizures.

Thyroglobulin may be used as a tumour marker for carcinoma of the thyroid.

Paraquat is extremely toxic and only small amounts of the order of 2–3 g may be fatal. High concentrations of oxygen enhance paraquat toxicity.

Rheumatoid factor is an IgM and it is present in a small but significant proportion of the healthy population.

The half-life of carboxyhaemoglobin is decreased by high concentrations of oxygen.

2. a.**T** b.**T** c.**T** d.**T** e.**F**

The short dexamethasone test may be abnormal with failure of cortisol suppression in patients with endogenous depression, alcoholism, dementia and anorexia as well as in Cushing's disease. Failure of suppression of serum cortisol concentrations during the short dexamethasone test might therefore be a problem in the differentiation of alcoholic pseudocushing's from Cushing's disease. The short dexamethasone test is useful in excluding Cushing's in patients with simple obesity who form the main differential diagnosis.

3. a.**T** b.**T** c.**T** d.**T** e.**F**

Cholecalciferol is converted to the active dihydroxycholecalciferol (vitamin D) through two hydroxylation steps, one in the liver and one in the kidneys. A suprising number of hormones may stimulate this hydroxylation, including parathyroid hormone. These hormones include growth hormone, cortisol, oestradiol and prolactin but not thyroxine.

4. a.**F** b.**T** c.**F** d.**T** e.**F**

Ethanol induces a wide range of metabolic changes when

regularly consumed. The toxicity of carbon tetrachloride is therefore enhanced by alcohol.

Alcohol and acetaldehyde can damage mitochondria through the direct inhibition of oxidative phosphorylation.

Alcohol dehydrogenase is a cytosolic enzyme.

The hypogonadism is due to increased testosterone conversion to oestradiol.

The metabolism of ethanol produces a decrease in the NAD^+: NADH ratio or an increase in the $NADH:NAD^+$ ratio. Excess NADH in the cytosol favours the production of lactate from pyruvate.

---

5. a.**T**　b.**T**　c.**T**　d.**T**　e.**T**

The syndrome of inappropriate antidiuresis may be associated with any of the patterns described, thereby making the measurement of AVP(ADH) of no value in the diagnosis of this condition. An inappropriately dilute serum osmolality in conjunction with an inappropriately concentrated urine is required to make the diagnosis. Conditions which may also result in difficulty in excreting a water load must be excluded at the same time.

---

6. a.**3**　b.**5**　c.**1**　d.**4**　e.**2**

Thiamine deficiency occurs particularly in alcoholics who drink spirits and results in Wernicke's encephalopathy and Korsakoff's psychosis. Vitamin C deficiency results in scurvy with subperiosteal haemorrhages, bleeding gums and loss of teeth. Niacin deficiency results in pellagra, which can present with angular stomatitis, diarrhoea, raw beef tongue, erythema and mental changes. Excessive intake of vitamin A and vitamin D may both be harmful. Both vitamins are available in over-the-counter preparations. An excessive intake of vitamin A may result in liver damage. It has been demonstrated that folic acid supplements may reduce the incidence of neural tube defects in pregnancy.

---

7. a.**5**　b.**3**　c.**4**　d.**1**　e.**2**

Aluminium in dialysis fluid may result in dialysis encephalopathy. In lead poisoning a blue line may be seen around the gums. Cadmium vapour poisoning, which may arise during industrial processes, results in lung and kidney damage. Cadmium is retained in the body following poisoning and its elimination may be followed by urine cadmium levels. Kidney damage due to cadmium poisoning may be monitored by urine β_2-microglobulin measurement. Mercury poisoning causes muscle tremor, irritability and salivation, as well as mental changes. Hat makers used to be susceptible to this form of poisoning and this contributes to the character of the 'mad hatter' in *Alice in Wonderland*. Selenium poisoning may occur in areas with soil rich in selenium and a diet rich in vegetables, such as some parts of China. Chronic selenium poisoning produces gastrointestinal symptoms and a garlic-like odour along with dry brittle hair.

---

8. a.**4**　b.**1**　c.**5**　d.**3**　e.**2**

Porphyria cutanea tarda is associated with increased hepatic iron stores; erythropoietic protoporphyria with photosensitivity. Acute intermittent porphyria causes an increased excretion of porphobilinogen in the urine which is used to screen for this condition. Variegate porphyria is associated with a deficiency of protoporphyrinogen oxidase. Lead poisoning, which is sometimes in the differential diagnosis of acute intermittent porphyria, is associated with increased urinary 5-aminolaevulinate (ALA) and erythrocyte zinc protoporphyrin.

---

9. a.**4**　b.**3**　c.**5**　d.**1**　e.**2**

Carbohydrate-deficient transferrin has been identified as a more specific marker for alcoholic liver disease than gamma-glutamyl transferase activity. Caeruloplasmin is an acute-phase reactant. In older LH assays where there was crossreaction between the LH β-subunit and the β-subunit of HCG, high LH values found by chance in samples from young women might indicate pregnancy. In modern assays this crossreactivity is eliminated and therefore suppressed LH and FSH levels in young women not on the oral contraceptive pill may indicate pregnancy. The 'triple test' used to screen for Down's syndrome usually comprises maternal age, α-FP and total HCG or free β-HCG. In some centres oestriol is also included. α-Fetoprotein in conjunction with HCG is also used in the monitoring of the treatment of some germ cell malignances.

10. a.**2**   b.**1**   c.**4**   d.**5**   e.**3**

Gilbert's syndrome is the commonest 'abnormality' of bilirubin metabolism, occurring in up to 7% of the population. Mildly raised unconjugated bilirubin levels are found on fasting or with intercurrent illness but jaundice is rarely seen. Urinary bilirubin pigment excretion is usually normal. In a haemolytic anaemia the transport of unconjugated bilirubin from haemolysed red blood cells to the liver exceeds the rate at which it can be conjugated and an unconjugated hyperbilirubinaemia occurs with increased urinary urobilinogen as there is no obstruction to bile flow. In obstructive jaundice there is a conjugated hyperbilirubinaemia as there is no defect in the glucuronidation enzyme system. As biliary flow is obstructed, there is a reduced production of urobilinogen in the gut and therefore absorption and excretion in the urine. In the Crigler–Najjar syndrome, which is usually fatal early in life, there is an unconjugated hyperbilirubinaemia and an absence of urinary urobilinogen, in contrast with the Dubin–Johnson syndrome where there is a conjugated hyperbilirubinaemia with normal or decreased level of urobilinogen in the urine.

11. a.**F**   b.**T**   c.**F**   d.**T**   e.**T**

While it is true that creatinine is secreted and reabsorbed to some extent in the normal kidney, creatinine excretion increases initially during the development of chronic renal failure and the accuracy of the creatinine clearance test decreases. Studies have shown that serial measurement of creatinine in serum may be as good a method of assessing deterioration in renal function as measuring creatinine clearance. Creatinine clearance may be affected by vigorous exercise during the collection period or a high dietary intake of protein. An assessment of 24-h urine creatinine excretion may be of use in determining whether the collection is complete as this is mainly dependent on muscle bulk. In macroamylasaemia, circulating amylase is bound to other proteins which means that it is not filtered as easily at the glomerulus. Urine excretion of amylase is therefore not increased despite the increased activity of amylase in the serum.

12. a.**T** b.**F** c.**T** d.**T** e.**T**

Adults may have sweat sodium values greater than the upper limit of normal for children. Due to the expertise required for the Gibson and Cooke iontophoresis method, it is rarely possible to firmly establish the diagnosis by this test alone especially as genetic markers are available. The cystic fibrosis gene is an autosomal recessive gene. Immunoreactive trypsin measurement in blood spots from neonates is another method of screening for cystic fibrosis. The defect in cystic fibrosis results in impaired chloride ion transport across cell membranes.

13. a.**T** b.**F** c.**T** d.**T** e.**T**

Phaeochromocytoma is thought to be present in approximately 0.5% of hypertensive patients; 10% of cases may be familial. Phaeochromocytoma occurs in association with MEN type II. Postural hypotension can occur in patients with the familial variant of phaeochromocytoma.

Bananas contain vanilla which is metabolized to substances which will interfere in measurement of urine NMA.

14. a.**T** b.**T** c.**F** d.**T** e.**T**

The mean serum concentration of 17-hydroxyprogesterone rises three-fold by 40 weeks, while the mean concentration of testosterone also increases slightly during pregnancy but the free androgen index falls due to increased binding protein. Serum prolactin levels rise to 3000 IU/l or more during pregnancy and may fall slowly after delivery if the mother breast-feeds. After the first 5–6 weeks of pregnancy, the major source of oestrogens is the placenta which converts fetal and maternal DHEAS to oestradiol.

15. a.**T** b.**F** c.**T** d.**F** e.**T**

The 6-min C-peptide response to 1 mg of IV glucagon may be used as a test of insulin reserve. Macroamylasaemia does not indicate anything other than circulating macrocomplexes of amylase and other proteins which prolong its half-life and therefore produce spuriously raised serum concentrations of amylase. Raised pleural fluid amylase concentrations greater than serum amylase concentrations may be found in patients with pancreatic pseudocyst. Serum lipase is as useful as amylase for the detection of acute pancreatitis. The glucagon test has also been advocated for the detection of insulinoma.

---

16. a.**F** b.**F** c.**F** d.**F** e.**T**

In the sick euthyroid syndrome thyroxine levels are subnormal while the TSH is in the reference range. TSH levels which are either completely suppressed below or just below the reference range are found in Graves' disease, viral thyroiditis, old age and hypopituitarism.

---

17. a.**F** b.**T** c.**F** d.**F** e.**T**

The absence of a raised serum uric acid concentration does not exclude gout. Uric acid has antioxidant properties and, with its relatively high concentration in plasma, must be one of the major contributors to the total antioxidant activity in plasma. In the Lesch–Nyhan syndrome there is a deficiency of the HGPRTase enzyme and resultant overproduction of uric acid. The measurement of urinary urate excretion may be of value as individuals with a raised urate level and a low excretion rate may benefit from uricosuric agents, while those with a high excretion rate may benefit more from allopurinol. Uric acid crystals may be deposited in other tissues and cause severe inflammation.

---

18. a.**F** b.**F** c.**F** d.**T** e.**F**

Hyponatraemia most commonly occurs in the clinical setting of a failure to excrete water and with the retention of sodium in addition to water but not in the same proportion, resulting in an expanded extracellular fluid volume and possibly oedema such as is found in left ventricular failure.

---

19. a.**F** b.**T** c.**T** d.**T** e.**T**

Polycystic ovary syndrome is associated with a raised LH:FSH ratio, which may be greater than 2.5. Mildly raised testosterone concentrations may be found but are not present in all individuals with this condition. Hirsutism and infertility as well as androgenic alopecia may be associated with this condition.

20. a.F   b.T   c.T   d.T   e.T

α_1-Antitrypsin deficiency by itself is not always sufficient to cause emphysema as cigarette smoking and atmospheric pollution also appear to contribute to its development. α_1-Antitrypsin functions as an elastase inhibitor. Deficiency may also be associated with cystic liver disease in children. Screening of the family of affected individuals is important as avoidance of cigarette smoking may reduce the likelihood of the development of emphysema.

21.

    a. Respiratory acidosis (5)
    b. Respiratory alkalosis (4)
    c. Metabolic acidosis (3)
    d. Metabolic alkalosis (1)
    e. Venous blood (2)

22.

    a. Gilbert's syndrome (2)
    b. Viral hepatitis (3)
    c. Hepatic metastases (5)
    d. End-stage cirrhosis (4)
    e. Primary biliary cirrhosis (1)

23.

    a. Poor compliance with treatment (3)
    b. Sick euthyroid syndrome (4)
    c. Adequate replacement (5)
    d. Euthyroid asymptomatic (1)
    e. Increased thyroxine-binding globulin (2)

24. a.T   b.T   c.T   d.F   e.T

Hypocalcaemia without hyperphosphataemia may occur with frusemide treatment, transfusion of citrated blood, medullary carcinoma of the thyroid and magnesium deficiency.

25. a.F   b.F   c.F   d.T   e.F

Raised concentrations of serum lactate dehydrogenase may be

found in patients with congestive cardiac failure due to hepatic congestion and in pernicious anaemia due to the fragility of the abnormal RBCs. In hypothyroidism raised concentrations of both creatine kinase and lactate dehydrogenase activity may be found in untreated patients, while raised lactate dehydrogenase in serum is also found in association with legionnaire's disease and *pneumocystis carinii* pneumonia associated with HIV infection.

---

26. a.**F** b.**F** c.**F** d.**F** e.**T**

---

27. a.**F** b.**F** c.**T** d.**F** e.**F**

A raised 1-h glucose value by itself does not confirm the diagnosis of diabetes mellitus. The WHO (1997) criteria for the diagnosis of diabetes mellitus state that the fasting venous glucose level must be greater than 7.8 mmol/l and/or the 2-h glucose level must be greater than 11.2 mmol/l to make the diagnosis. The correct timing of the 2-h glucose value is essential for the correct interpretation of this test. A standard glucose tolerance test cannot be used to exclude reactive hypoglycaemia and measurement of glycosylated haemoglobin is not yet accepted as a substitute for a glucose tolerance test.

---

28. a.**F** b.**F** c.**T** d.**F** e.**F**

Multiple myeloma may cause a pseudohyponatraemia if sodium concentrations are measured by flame photometry or by an indirect ion-selective electrode. Excessive water consumption and treatment with DDAVP may result in hyponatraemia. Overtreatment with potassium-sparing diuretics may cause hyponatraemia due to salt loss. A low-salt diet rarely causes hyponatraemia as the kidneys are extremely efficient at conserving sodium. Treatment with carbamazepine may cause hyponatraemia due to the syndrome of inappropriate antidiuresis.

---

29. a.**T** b.**T** c.**F** d.**F** e.**T**

Mild hypercalcaemia may sometimes occur with Addison's disease and thiazide diuretic administration. Hypercalcaemia is said to occur in patients with Paget's disease who are immobilized.

30. a.T b.T c.F d.F e.F

Hypokalaemia occurs in theophylline overdose and also in association with marked hypercalcaemia due to sodium loss and exchange of potassium for sodium in the distal renal tubule. Treatment with an ACE inhibitor may cause hyperkalaemia, particularly in the elderly.

31. a.5 b.4 c.2 d.3 e.1

The increased metabolic rate of thyrotoxic patients may produce low fructosamine concentrations due to increased turnover of protein. The ketones, acetoacetate and β-hydroxybutyrate produced in diabetic ketoacidosis interfere with creatinine measurement, producing falsely raised values. Treatment of temporal arteritis with prednisolone will interfere with cortisol measurement as prednisolone interferes in the cortisol assay. In rheumatoid arthritis increased platelet fragility, which causes platelet lysis when blood clots, can produce a pseudohyperkalaemia. In patients with liver failure or renal failure and also neonates and pregnant women, digoxin-like immunoreactive substances are produced and these can interfere with digoxin measurement.

32. a.F b.F c.F d.F e.T

All the listed biochemical results with the exception of a suppressed plasma ACTH concentration may occur in Addison's disease.

33. a.F b.F c.F d.F e.T

All the listed biochemical abnormalities may occur in patients with hypothyroidism with the exception of hypocalcaemia, unless the patient has hypothyroidism as a result of a partial thyroidectomy which has also removed the parathyroid glands.

34. a.F b.T c.T d.T e.F

Ketoacidosis occurs during starvation and may occur during alcoholic intoxication and salicylate poisoning.

35. a.5   b.4   c.1   d.3   e.2

Hypomagnesaemia may cause hypoparathyroidism. Chronic hypocalcaemia causes stellate cataracts. Treatment with cisplatinum may cause hypophosphataemia. Hyperglycaemia in patients with diabetes mellitus may result in hyponatraemia due to movement of water from within cells to the interstitial space, thereby producing a dilutional hyponatraemia. The use of purgatives may result in hypokalaemia. In the ITU hypophosphataemia may result in difficulty weaning patients off the ventilator as it causes weakness of the diaphragmatic muscles.

36. a.F   b.T   c.T   d.F   e.F

17α-OH progesterone levels would be of use in excluding mild or late-onset congenital adrenal hyperplasia, while the LH:FSH ratio would be useful in identifying the polycystic ovarian syndrome and the testosterone level would be of value in establishing androgen excess. A single serum cortisol concentration would be of little value due to the diurnal rhythm of cortisol and the possibility of normal morning cortisol levels with the loss of diurnal rhythm not being detected in early Cushing's syndrome. A sex hormone-binding globulin concentration would probably be of little help but could be used to calculate the free androgen index.

37. a.F   b.F   c.F   d.T   e.F

Urinary retention causes a marked increase in PSA levels as does prostatitis and prostatic biopsy. Minor rises in PSA levels can also occur with BPH. The other statements are incorrect, as 'normal' PSA values rise with age and occasionally measurable PSA values may be found in women. Digital rectal examination has not been proved to cause an increase in PSA levels unless examination also includes a biopsy. Due to false positives, PSA is not suitable as a screening test for the general population in the detection of prostate neoplasm.

38. a.F   b.F   c.F   d.T   e.F

Cholesterol concentrations fluctuate but not in a diurnal pattern while cortisol, zinc, TSH and bilirubin concentrations do show a diurnal pattern. Zinc concentrations in plasma may be below the 'normal' range during the afternoon.

---

39. a.**F**   b.**F**   c.**F**   d.**F**   e.**T**

The mean cholesterol concentration in patients presenting with premature coronary artery disease is close to the average cholesterol concentration in the population at 6.3 mmol/l. Serum cholesterol concentrations are higher in the winter than the summer. The optimal time for measuring cholesterol concentration following a myocardial infarction is on admission to hospital, as most patients do not have their cholesterol checked when reviewed at 3 months. Raised triglycerides alone may indicate increased risk of IHD as high triglycerides indicate LDL subclass pattern B which is more atherogenic. Optimally, the cholesterol concentration ought to be measured four times before treatment is instituted in order to assess the limits within which an individual's cholesterol concentration fluctuates.

---

40. a.**F**   b.**T**   c.**F**   d.**F**   e.**F**

The best single measurement to assess thyroid function is serum TSH measurement.

---

41. a.**T**   b.**F**   c.**F**   d.**T**   e.**T**

Raised serum prolactin levels persist in the postpartum period especially if the mother breastfeeds her child. Serum prolactin levels of 1000 IU/l or more can be produced by stress and some medication. Not all patients with raised serum prolactin concentrations have galactorrhoea. Serum prolactin levels fall on resting and cannulated prolactin levels collected while a patient is resting in hospital may be useful in identifying individuals with raised levels due to stress. Raised prolactin levels may also occur with big prolactin as this has a longer half-life.

---

42. a.**F**   b.**T**   c.**T**   d.**T**   e.**F**

A CKMB percentage greater than 20% is suggestive of a macro-CK. While myoglobin is not cardiospecific, it rises early during myocardial infarction and has been used as a marker for this. Raised serum ferritin concentrations occur in haemochromatosis. The other statements are true.

43. a.**T** b.**T** c.**T** d.**T** e.**T**

None of the statements are untrue.

44. a.**T** b.**F** c.**F** d.**T** e.**F**

In adults, growth hormone levels gradually decline with age. A single raised growth hormone level is not diagnostic of acromegaly. Stress causes growth hormone levels to rise while hyperglycaemia will suppress growth hormone levels. In children the growth hormone response to exercise is of use in excluding growth hormone deficiency. In adults and children growth hormone levels tend to fluctuate throughout the day.

45. a.**T** b.**T** c.**F** d.**F** e.**T**

Raised Lp(a) concentrations, triglyceride concentrations and fibrinogen concentrations are independent risk factors for premature coronary artery disease. LDL subclass patterns may be of importance in the development of coronary artery disease, as might be deficiency of antioxidants such as vitamin C and vitamin E, but these factors have not yet been established as independent risk factors although there is evidence that they are of importance in developing coronary artery disease.

46. a.**5** b.**4** c.**2** d.**3** e.**1**

47. a.**F** b.**F** c.**F** d.**T** e.**T**

The specificity of a test is the percent negativity in the absence of disease. The sensitivity of a test is the percent positivity in the presence of disease. The prevalence of a disease is the number of subjects with the disease per 100 000 population. The incidence of a disease is the number of new cases per year per 100 000 population. The receiver operator characteristic curve demonstrates the sensitivity and specificity of a test depending on the prevalence of the disease in the population studied.

48. a.**T** b.**T** c.**F** d.**F** e.**T**

If the albumin concentration in serum is used as a nutritional marker then approximately 50% of patients in surgical wards are undernourished. Serum albumin concentrations are a poor marker of nutritional status in these circumstances. When patients are euglycaemic prior to commencement of a standard parenteral nutrition regimen, it is unlikely that they will become hyperglycaemic as a complication of TPN. Patients in hospital who have had an operation do not have an overall increased calorie need compared to preoperative patients. While their BMR may be increased, they are less active and as a result their total calorie need per 24 h remains around 2000 kcal/day. If parenteral feeding is to be given for a short supportive period only, then trace elements and essential fatty acids are not necessarily part of the regimen. Glutamine supplements during TPN help maintain bowel function.

---

49. a.**T**   b.**T**   c.**T**   d.**F**   e.**F**

Serum CA 125 levels may be raised in patients with a range of intraabdominal conditions including ascites. Marginally raised levels may be found in endometriosis. CA 153 may be raised in breast carcinoma and also liver disease, tuberculosis or SLE. Raised α-FP levels may occur with alcoholic hepatitis or viral hepatitis as well as hepatoma. CEA concentrations may be raised by renal failure.

---

50. a.**F**   b.**F**   c.**F**   d.**T**   e.**T**

Serum troponin T levels may be raised following any injury to the heart. A single measurement of troponin T more than 12 h after onset of chest pain is sufficient to confirm a MI. Less than 12 h after the onset of chest pain, troponin T levels may be normal even in individuals having a myocardial infarction. A raised troponin T level in individuals with angina indicates a poorer prognosis and levels may remain raised for up to 2 weeks.

Haematology

51. Causes of a raised MCV:

    a. Aplastic anaemia
    b. Myelodysplasia
    c. Inherited sideroblastic anaemia
    d. G6PD deficiency in haemolytic phase
    e. Pregnancy

52. Part two of the Schilling test corrects in the following conditions:

    a. Crohn's disease
    b. Anatomical blind loop
    c. Partial gastrectomy
    d. Pernicious anaemia with high levels of intrinsic factor antibody secretion in the gut
    e. Tropical sprue

53. Peripheral blood features of megaloblastic anaemia include:

    a. Hypersegmented neutrophils
    b. Poikilocytosis
    c. Basophilic stippling
    d. Target cells
    e. Erythrocyte fragmentation

54. Causes of folate deficiency are:

    a. Congestive heart failure
    b. Haemodialysis
    c. Myelosclerosis
    d. Non-Hodgkin's lymphoma
    e. Ileocolic fistula

55. Regarding folate metabolism:

    a. Total body store is 10 mg
    b. Daily adult requirement is 10 µg
    c. The monoglutamate form is commonest in food
    d. The vitamin is highly heat sensitive
    e. Absorption occurs rapidly in the jejunum

56. Iron absorption is improved by:

   a. Pregnancy
   b. Ferric state
   c. Iron in the haem form
   d. Phytates
   e. Protein

57. Iron deficiency may be associated with:

   a. A normal MCV
   b. A lowered zinc protoporphyrin
   c. Increased rate of bacterial infection
   d. Atrophic gastritis
   e. Peripheral neuropathy

58. In healthy iron metabolism:

   a. The body store is 8 g
   b. Daily absorption is 10 mg
   c. Red cell haemoglobin constitutes most of the body's iron
   d. Iron within haem binds directly to oxygen
   e. Siderocytes are common in iron-deficient erythroblasts

59. Causes of resistance to erythropoietin therapy:

   a. Aluminium toxicity
   b. Iron overload
   c. Blood loss
   d. Haemolysis
   e. Infection

60. Potential complications of erythropoietin therapy:

   a. Hypocalcaemia
   b. Hypertension
   c. Arteriovenous fistula thrombosis
   d. Seizures
   e. Depression

61. Causes of cold-type autoimmune haemolytic anaemia include:

   a. Non-Hodgkin's lymphoma
   b. Chronic granulocytic leukaemia

c. *Mycoplasma pneumoniae*
d. Pneumococcal pneumonia
e. Childhood measles

62. Causes of warm autoimmune haemolytic anaemia include:

a. Non-Hodgkin's lymphoma
b. L-dopa therapy
c. Bronchial carcinoma
d. Rheumatoid arthritis
e. SLE

63. Causes of non-immune acquired haemolytic anaemia include:

a. Malaria
b. Drowning
c. Paroxysmal nocturnal haemoglobinuria
d. Gram-negative sepsis
e. Acute myeloid leukaemia

64. Causes of microangiopathic haemolytic anaemia include:

a. Thrombotic thrombocytopenic purpura
b. Carcinomatosis
c. Systemic lupus erythematosus
d. Uterine fibroids
e. Cardiac valve prosthesis

65. Causes of oxidative haemolysis include:

a. Chlorate
b. Phenylbutazone
c. Dapsone
d. Amylnitrate
e. Salazopyrin

66. Paroxysmal cold haemoglobinuria:

a. Often presents with abdominal pain and haemoglobinuria
b. Is associated with primary syphilis
c. May follow childhood viral infection
d. Is associated with a positive Donath–Landsteiner antibody
e. Usually produces life-threatening haemolysis

67. The direct Coombs test is:

    a. Positive in paroxysmal nocturnal haemoglobinuria
    b. Positive in paroxysmal cold haemoglobinuria
    c. Negative in Evans syndrome
    d. Positive in meningococcal microangiopathic haemolysis
    e. Positive in the haemolytic uraemic syndrome

68. Paroxysmal nocturnal haemoglobinuria is associated with:

    a. Severe bleeding tendency
    b. Haemolysis
    c. Pancytopenia
    d. Resistance to complement-mediated haemolysis
    e. Transformation to acute lymphoblastic leukaemia

69. Hereditary spherocytosis is associated with:

    a. A recessive inheritance
    b. A variable degree of spherocytosis on the blood film
    c. Increased red cell fragility which corrects following 24 h incubation at 37°C
    d. Positive autohaemolysis test which is glucose dependent
    e. Reduced erythrocyte content of spectrin

70. Clinical features of hereditary spherocytosis include:

    a. Gall stones
    b. Renal stones
    c. Failure to thrive
    d. Leg ulcers
    e. Aplastic crisis

71. G6PD deficiency is:

    a. An autosomally inherited disorder
    b. Commonest in Africa
    c. Usually due to genetic deletion
    d. Associated with sensitivity to chloraquine
    e. A cause of persistent neonatal jaundice

72. G6PD deficiency is:

    a. Diagnosed on a blood film

b. A cause of abdominal pain and haemoglobinuria
c. Problematic in heterozygous individuals
d. Associated with folate deficiency
e. Associated with many different genetic aberrations

---

73. Homozygous sickle cell anaemia:

a. Results from a variable point mutation
b. Confers protection from malaria
c. Responds to splenectomy
d. Is associated with a degenerative retinopathy
e. Can produce rapidly fatal splenic sequestration in children

---

74. In sickle cell anaemia:

a. Exchange blood transfusion is routine management
b. Bone marrow transplantation is a suitable option for most adults
c. Surgery should only be performed once the HbS level is below 50%
d. Penicillin prophylaxis is widely recommended
e. Leg ulcers are a feature

---

75. Haemoglobin C disease:

a. Results from a substitution of the sixth amino acid in β-globin
b. Usually produces severe anaemia in the homozygous state
c. May be inherited coincident with haemoglobin S
d. Produces plentiful target cells on the blood film
e. Produces a haemoglobin band that runs with haemoglobin A on cellulose acetate electrophoresis

---

76. In chronic myeloid leukaemia:

a. Visual symptoms are a frequent presenting feature
b. The blast count is usually >10% in the marrow
c. The Philadelphia translocation is between chromosomes 9 and 21
d. Autologous marrow transplantation is often curative
e. Chronic phase usually lasts >8 years

77. β-Thalassaemia trait:

    a. Is a cause of macrocytosis
    b. Results in a raised red cell count
    c. Is usually asymptomatic
    d. May have a slightly raised haemoglobin F
    e. May feature target cells in the blood film

78. In adult acute myeloid leukaemia:

    a. Chemotherapy produces remission in less than 50% of cases
    b. Splenomegaly is not uncommon
    c. Thrombocytopenia is frequent
    d. Occurrence is most common < 40 years of age
    e. Allogeneic marrow transplantation offers the best long-term cure

79. Microcytic anaemia may occur in:

    a. Folate deficiency
    b. β-Thalassaemia major
    c. Homozygous sickle disease
    d. Rheumatoid arthritis
    e. Coeliac disease

80. Haemophilia A is associated with:

    a. Chronic joint disease
    b. A prolonged prothrombin time
    c. A low fibrinogen level
    d. Spontaneous cerebral haemorrhage
    e. Frequent gum bleeding following brushing

81. Neutropenia is a feature of:

    a. Acute leukaemia
    b. Steroid therapy
    c. Pregnancy
    d. Thalassaemia
    e. Viral infection

82. Activated protein C resistance:

    a. Is the commonest form of inherited thrombophilia

b. Is due to activated factor 8 being resistant to activated protein C
c. Occurs in 5% of healthy controls
d. Analysis of the gene for factor 5 is the most specific way to make the diagnosis
e. Is commoner in men

---

83. Features of hyposplenism are common in:

a. Coeliac disease
b. Thalassaemia major
c. Sickle cell trait
d. Amyloidosis affecting the spleen
e. Gaucher's disease

---

84. The following agents are well-recognized causes of aplastic anaemia:

a. Phenytoin
b. Interferon-α
c. Septrin
d. Chlorpromazine
e. Cimetidine

---

85. Side effects associated with the administration of antilymphocyte globulin are:

a. Peripheral thrombophlebitis
b. Thrombocytopenia
c. ARDS
d. Glomerulonephritis
e. Proteinuria

---

86. The following conditions have been associated with the presentation of bone marrow hypoplasia:

a. Paroxysmal nocturnal haemoglobinuria
b. Acute lymphoblastic leukaemia
c. Fanconi's anaemia
d. Massive blood transfusion reaction
e. Blackfan–Diamond syndrome

87. With regards to the genetics of haemoglobin formation:

    a. Chromosone 16 contains two active genes for the α-globin chain

    b. Chromosone 11 contains two active genes for the β-globin chain

    c. There are two pseudogenes for the α-globin chain on chromosome 16

    d. HbF is comprised of two α chains and two δ chains

    e. HbH consists of tetramers of the β chain

88. Homozygous sickle cell disease:

    a. Has cold as one of the most important precipitating causes of crisis

    b. Produces no HbA on electrophoresis

    c. Produces a microcytic anaemia

    d. Results from valine replacing glutamic acid at the sixth amino acid in the β-globin chain

    e. Produces a normal red cell lifespan

89. In chronic lymphatic leukaemia:

    a. Haemolytic anaemia occurs in 50% of cases

    b. Hyperleucocytosis is frequently problematic

    c. The characteristic cell phenotype is CD 19+15+

    d. Immunoglobulin levels are often decreased

    e. A monoclonal gammopathy occurs in up to 10%

90. In primary proliferative polycythaemia:

    a. The plasma volume is usually normal

    b. The red cell mass may be normal (at diagnosis)

    c. Venesection remains the treatment of choice for most patients

    d. Splenomegaly is usually present

    e. Erythrocyte colonies can grow in vitro without the support of erythropoietin

91. Homozygous β-thalassaemia:

    a. Is most commonly treated with a blood transfusion regimen plus desferrioxamine

    b. Is associated with leg ulcers

c. May give rise to pseudotumours
d. Produces a microcytic hypochromic anaemia
e. Results in HbF as the predominant band on haemoglobin electrophoresis

---

92. The β-thalassaemia mutation:

a. Is usually a gene deletion
b. Has over 50 different genetic defects
c. Confers relative protection against malaria in the homozygous form
d. Results in a reduction or absence of β-globin synthesis
e. Is the only cause of a raised HbA2

---

93. With regard to β-thalassaemia:

a. Bone marrow transplantation in childhood is a potential management option
b. Hormone replacement is nearly always effective in the homozygous state
c. Splenectomy does have a place in the management of the homozygous state
d. Oral iron chelators are now becoming available
e. Blood transfusion regimens should only be considered late in the management of homozygous children

---

94. With regard to low molecular weight heparin:

a. LMW heparin crosses the placenta but unfractionated heparin does not
b. LMW heparin is licensed in pregnancy
c. LMW heparin is superior to unfractionated heparin in prophylaxis in orthopaedic surgery
d. LMW heparin is superior to unfractionated heparin in prophylaxis in general surgery
e. LMW heparin has equivalent antithrombin properties to unfractionated heparin

95. Heparin-induced thrombocytopenia:

   a. Occurs equally as commonly with unfractionated as low molecular weight heparin
   b. Occurs in 10% of people treated with heparin
   c. Can be associated with new thromboembolic events
   d. Has a 30% mortality
   e. May be treated by substituting low molecular weight heparin for unfractionated heparin

96. With regard to warfarin:

   a. It reduces posttranslational γ-carboxylation of glutamic acid residues in vitamin K-dependent proteins
   b. It potentiates vitamin K reductase
   c. PIVKAs in themselves have an inhibitory effect on the clotting mechanism
   d. Warfarin causes factor 10 levels to fall before factor 7 levels
   e. It passes readily into breast milk

97. Warfarin interactions:

   a. NSAIDs prolong the INR by displacing warfarin from carrier protein
   b. Tricyclic antidepressants prolong the INR by suppressing hepatic microenzyme activity
   c. Phenytoin prolongs the INR by inducing hepatic enzyme activity
   d. Antibiotics increase vitamin K absorption
   e. Thyroxine therapy prolongs the INR by altering the hepatic receptor for warfarin

98. Antithrombin 3 deficiency:

   a. Is inherited in an autosomal recessive manner
   b. Accounts for 20% of people who have recurrent thromboembolism
   c. May produce heparin resistance
   d. Merits prophylactic anticoagulation even in individuals who have not had a thromboembolic event
   e. Merits some form of prophylactic anticoagulation during pregnancy

99. Antithrombin 3 deficiency:

a. Produces more venous than arterial thromboses
b. Usually results from gene insertion or deletion of one or more nucleotides
c. Is the commonest inherited deficiency of the naturally occurring anticoagulants
d. Can manifest in the heterozygous from
e. May manifest as a functional deficiency of the protein although antigen levels of the protein may be normal

100. Protein C deficiency:

a. Is equally bad in its homozygous and heterozygous forms
b. Produces equal amounts of venous and arterial thromboses
c. Can produce hazardous warfarinization
d. Is inherited as an autosomal dominant
e. Can be acquired in renal failure

---

51. a.**T** b.**T** c.**F** d.**T** e.**T**

The MCV tends to drift upwards in aplastic anaemia and myelodysplasia; this seems to be a reflection of the changes in erythropoiesis rather than any vitamin deficiency. Inherited sideroblastic anaemia tends to have a low MCV with a dimorphic blood picture, whereas acquired sideroblastic anaemia as part of myelodysplasia tends to have a raised MCV.

During any form of haemolysis an increased reticulocyte count will elevate the MCV.

Pregnancy puts up the MCV and this seems to be independent of any vitamin deficiency.

---

52. a.**F** b.**F** c.**T** d.**F** e.**F**

The Schilling test was often performed in two stages. The fashion now is to perform a Dicopac procedure, where the B12 is given orally as two different types of cobalt isotope, one being attached to intrinsic factor. In the classic part two Schilling test, the B12 isotope is also given with intrinsic factor.

Obviously, in intrinsic intestinal disease such as Crohn's disease and tropical sprue the addition of intrinsic factor in the test does not improve B12 absorption. In the presence of an anatomical blind loop, oral vitamin B12 tends to be metabolized by the organisms contained therein, thus stopping the B12 getting to the site of absorption; the presence of intrinsic factor does not correct this. Occasionally patients with pernicious anaemia may secrete large amounts of antibody to intrinsic factor into the gut. This can be a binding or blocking type of IF antibody but occasionally it can interfere with the classic part two Schilling test, correction for pernicious anaemia.

---

53. a.**T** b.**T** c.**T** d.**F** e.**T**

Hypersegmented neutrophils are a classic feature of megaloblastic anaemia and are due to the right-shifted nature of the process. Because of the abnormalities in erythropoiesis within the marrow, a certain amount of red cell breakdown and destruction occurs there and in the spleen. Poikilocytosis and fragmentation are therefore common and can be very marked in advanced megaloblastic change. Basophilic stippling is a well-recognized feature of megaloblastosis and is due to residual RNA. It is also a feature of thalassaemia major and minor, haemolysis, myelodysplasia, liver disease, lead poisoning, etc. (a common MRCP question). Target cells are not seen in megaloblastic anaemia but are a feature of liver disease, alcohol, haemoglobin C, obstructive jaundice, sickle cell disease, thalassaemia major and minor and iron deficiency anaemia.

---

54. a.T   b.T   c.T   d.T   e.F

Folate metabolism can be rapidly exhausted. Processes of haemolysis, malignancy and haemodialysis can all accelerate this. Patients with chronic haemolysis such as thalassaemia or sickle cell disease or myelosclerosis may require prophylactic folic acid. Similarly, folate replacement for people on haemodialysis is often given. Folate deficiency in congestive heart failure is due to increased consumption of folate and also a reduction in absorption. In ileocolic fistula, the increase in intestinal bacteria actually results in more folate being produced and absorbed.

---

55. a.T   b.F   c.F   d.T   e.T

The total body store of an average adult is about 10 mg of folate. About 100 µg of folate is lost each day due to shedding of cells, etc., therefore about 100 µg per day is the minimum replacement for this loss. Simple arithmetic demonstrates that this is about one-hundredth of the body store and it is not surprising therefore that this store can be depleted quite quickly.

The polyglutamate form is commonest in nature and this gets converted to the monoglutamate form during metabolism within the body but eventually within the cell the polyglutamate form is reconstituted. Overcooking vegetables depletes folic acid content so they should therefore be eaten al dente.

---

56. a.T   b.F   c.T   d.F   e.T

Under the circumstances of iron depletion the body takes corrective action to increase iron absorption from the gut. Pregnancy is one such instance. Iron in the haem form rather than in elemental form is also more rapidly absorbed, especially if it is in the presence of protein. It is the ferrous state rather than the ferric state that favours absorption. Phytates tend to bind to iron and reduce its absorption.

---

57. a.**T**   b.**F**   c.**F**   d.**T**   e.**F**

In the early stages of iron deficiency the MCV is normal. When there is insufficient iron for binding to the protoporphyrin part of the haem molecule, other elements such as zinc take its place. Therefore, increased amounts of zinc protoporphyrin (ZPP) in red cells indicate that there is a deficiency in iron. This test is very rapid and is probably as good if not better than ferritin; it is certainly superior to iron and TIBC.

Bacteria require iron for healthy growth. Therefore a deficiency of iron puts bacterial growth at a disadvantage. It has been argued that correcting iron deficiency in the tropics can actually *increase* bacterial infections. Mucosal atrophy in the oral cavity and the stomach are common features of iron deficiency; peripheral neutropathy is not.

---

58. a.**F**   b.**F**   c.**T**   d.**T**   e.**F**

The adult store of iron is about 4 g, most of which is found within circulating red cells. An average diet will provide about 10 mg of iron but only 1 mg of this is actually absorbed.

Within each haem molecule, six available valencies on the iron atom are bound as follows: four to the protoporphyrin ring, one to the globin chain and one is available for binding to oxygen.

Siderocytes are small cytoplasmic collections of iron seen commonly in maturing marrow erythroblasts as a normal feature; they are therefore not a common feature of iron deficiency. Sideroblasts, on the other hand, are pathological and the term refers to those maturing erythroblasts with iron-laden mitochondria surrounding their nucleus.

---

59. a.**T**   b.**F**   c.**T**   d.**T**   e.**T**

Aluminium toxicity and concurrent infection are common causes of erythropoietin resistance in renal failure.

Due to regular haemodialysis patients tend to become iron deficient which is another cause of erythropoietin resistance.

(Iron overload is very unusual in renal failure and most patients receive intravenous iron following haemodialysis to make up for iron loss.)

Ongoing haemolysis can occur during uraemia and this may outpace the ability of erythropoietin to stimulate erythropoiesis.

---

60. a.F   b.T   c.T   d.T   e.F

Over vigorous use of erythropoietin in uraemia did lead initially to increases in blood volume and viscosity that led to hypertension, thrombosis within fistulae and occasionally seizure. More judicious use of erythropoietin in renal failure can improve the haemoglobin sufficiently to dramatically improve clinical symptoms but without necessarily getting the haemoglobin into the normal range. Hyperkalaemia is also a recognized complication but hypocalcaemia is not. Depression is not a well-recognized complication.

---

61. a.T   b.F   c.T   d.F   e.T

The term cold haemolytic antibodies refers to those antibodies with properties allowing them to bind to red cells at temperatures below 37°C. This is obviously a laboratory rather than a clinical distinction. Such antibodies often bind to the I antigen on the red cell surface. These can be seen following infection such as mycoplasma and measles but not bacterial infections usually.

Chronic granulocytic leukaemia is not associated with any haemolytic process.

---

62. a.T   b.T   c.T   d.T   e.T

Non-Hodgkin's lymphoma can produce warm or cold haemolytic anaemia. Methyldopa as well as L-dopa stimulates autoantibodies which are usually warm in type. Inflammatory and malignant processes can also be associated with warm haemolytic anaemia.

---

63. a.T   b.T   c.T   d.T   e.F

Heavy malarial infestation of erythrocytes can lead to red cell destruction and an intravascular haemolysis. This manifests as blackwater fever in severe falciparum infections.

Hypotonic stress during drowning can lead to red cell disruption.

In PNH erythrocytes are extremely susceptible to complement lysis because they lack certain protective proteins (DAF). PNH is associated with an intravascular and non-antibody mediated haemolytic process which is Coomb's negative.

Severe bacterial infections including Gram-negative sepsis can result in DIC and microangiopathic haemolysis (other infections include meningococcus, pneumococcus, psittacosis and Yersinia).

AML is not associated with haemolytic anaemia.

---

64. a.**T** b.**T** c.**T** d.**F** e.**T**

In TTP large amounts of fibrin are laid down within the microvasculature. This causes red cell fragmentation as the cells try to negotiate these vessels. Carcinomatosis and vasculitic processes will also lead to microangiopathic haemolysis due to red cell disruption by fibrin deposition.

Uterine fibroids are not commonly associated with MAHA.

When prosthetic cardiac valves become dysfunctional they cause a lot of turbulence in the large vessels which can in turn result in red cell fragmentation.

---

65. a.**T** b.**F** c.**T** d.**T** e.**T**

Within the erythrocyte the pentose phosphate shunt (G6PD pathway) is the usual source of reduced glutathione which acts as an antioxidant within the cells. This process is deficient in G6PD deficiency. However, even in healthy individuals the process can be overwhelmed by certain oxidating chemicals or drugs such as chlorate, dapsone, amyl nitrate and salazopyrin. Phenylbutazone is not an oxidizing agent.

---

66. a.**T** b.**F** c.**T** d.**T** e.**F**

Following a drop in body temperature, the Donath–Landsteiner antibody binds to red cells and results in intravascular haemolysis. This manifests as haemoglobinuria. This is an unusual feature of tertiary and congenital syphilis, but it can also follow certain viral infections. Haemolysis is usually mild and very rarely causes a major problem. The Donath–Landsteiner antibody was described by these two pathologists who found that the antibody needed to be incubated with red cells below body temperature before haemolysis could occur in vitro.

---

67. a.**F** b.**T** c.**F** d.**F** e.**F**

In the direct Coombs test, animal sera that have been raised against human immunoglobulin are mixed with the patient's red cells. This is then spun down. If the red cells have human antibody on their surface, the animal antisera will cross-link these molecules and cause the red cells to agglutinate. Any process that is associated with antibodies upon the surface of red cells will therefore cause the direct Coombs test to be positive. In this question only paroxysmal cold haemoglobinuria and Evans syndrome are associated with antibodies on the red cell surface. All the other conditions are not.

---

68. a.**F** b.**T** c.**T** d.**F** e.**F**

In PNH cell surface membranes do not possess the molecular machinery to protect them against complement lysis. There is therefore a tendency to haemolysis when red cells become susceptible to complement lysis, i.e. when blood pH drops such as in sleep. This forms the basis of the Ham's test in the laboratory. PNH is associated with pancytopenia and can lead to acute myeloid leukaemia (transformation to ALL would be extremely unusual). Thrombocytopenia may be progressive but other than this there is not usually a severe bleeding tendency.

---

69. a.**T** b.**T** c.**F** d.**T** e.**F**

Hereditary spherocytosis is a mixture of different conditions which can either have recessive or dominant inheritance. The biochemical result is an abnormality within the spectrin molecule rather than a reduction in the amount of spectrin content. The number of spherocytes on the blood film can be very variable, from 2% up to 90+%. The red cell fragility usually worsens after incubation. When red cells are incubated in their own serum over 24 h there is a stress on their glycolytic pathway. This leads to more rapid haemolysis in HS compared to normal, but the addition of glucose to the incubation can partly correct this.

70. a.**T** b.**F** c.**T** d.**T** e.**T**

Increased haemolysis results in the formation of bilirubin stones rather than renal stones. If the patient is anaemic as a child, this may result in failure to thrive. Leg ulcers are a feature. Aplastic crises may occur when a parvovirus infection puts additional stress on the marrow, in particular erythropoiesis. Such a crisis normally corrects over a few weeks.

71. a.**F** b.**T** c.**F** d.**F** e.**T**

Deficiency of G6PD is very common in Africa and is an X-linked recessive disorder. A number of different point mutations have been described in this deficiency and it is not due to large genetic deletion. Chloroquine is relatively safe in this disorder but primaquine can precipitate haemolysis. Apart from acute haemolytic crisis, G6PD deficiency can also present as neonatal jaundice and a chronic haemolytic anaemia.

72. a.**F** b.**T** c.**F** d.**T** e.**T**

The diagnosis of G6PD deficiency can only be made on enzyme analysis; the blood film cannot confer a positive diagnosis although it will demonstrate features of haemolysis. Intravascular haemolysis may present as haemoglobinuria and abdominal pain. Heterozygous individuals, i.e. female carriers, are not normally symptomatic but occasionally can have a mild anaemia. It is important to screen prospective spouses for red cell problems. All patients with potential haemolysis should receive folate therapy, i.e. haemoglobinopathies as well as G6PD-deficient patients. There are many different point mutations described causing this genetic abnormality.

73. a.**F** b.**F** c.**F** d.**F** e.**T**

Unlike thalassaemias and G6PD deficiency, haemoglobin S results from the same genetic change in all patients (glutamic acid being replaced by valine at the sixth amino acid in the β chain). In the heterozygous state malarial infection will cause sickling within a cell and destruction of the cell plus parasite, therefore limiting the disease. However, in the homozygous state, malaria can be an overwhelming and lethal infection. Because patients get infarction within their spleen they tend to have autosplenectomy and elective splenectomy plays little part in the management of this disease. Due to retinal ischaemia patients can get a proliferative retinopathy rather than degenerative change. In children, the sickling process can become very rapid within the spleen, leading to sequestration and sudden and massive increase in splenic size which can be lethal. Parents are often taught to detect this by palpating the abdomen and, if worried, to bring the child to hospital rapidly.

---

74. a.**F**   b.**F**   c.**F**   d.**T**   e.**T**

Most patients with sickle cell anaemia are treated with supportive blood transfusion regularly. Exchange blood transfusion is a major undertaking and is only performed in unusual situations such as chest syndrome or priapism. Transplantation is performed occasionally but only in childhood. Sicklers may undergo a general anaesthetic but they have to have transfusion beforehand to dilute their haemoglobin S down to 20% of total. Some centres now advise that this is *not* always necessary. Due to autosplenectomy, penicillin V is given prophylactically. Leg ulcers are a common feature of sickle cell anaemia due to microvascular ischaemia.

---

75. a.**T**   b.**F**   c.**T**   d.**T**   e.**F**

The amino acid substitution is at the same position as in sickle cell anaemia (lycine replaces glutamic acid).

The homozygous and heterozygous states are associated with a mild degree of anaemia usually but with marked target cells on the blood film.

It is possible to inherit haemoglobin C on one chromosome 11 and haemoglobin S on the other chromosome 11 and therefore produce haemoglobin SC disease.

Haemoglobin C runs slowly and falls some way behind haemoglobin A.

---

76. a.**T**   b.**F**   c.**F**   d.**F**   e.**F**

Due to hyperleucocytosis, visual symptoms are quite common at presentation.

The majority of patients have a low blast count in the marrow at presentation.

The classic Philadelphia translocation is between chromosomes 9 and 22.

Allogeneic BMT is the only means of curing this disease although autologous BMT *may* improve survival.

Chronic phase lasts between 2 and 5 years prior to transformation.

---

77. a.F   b.T   c.T   d.T   e.T

β-Thalassaemia trait is a cause of microcytosis. The red cell count is usually raised. Most carriers are asymptomatic. Classically, the haemoglobin A2 is raised and the haemoglobin F is also occasionally raised. Target cells are usually seen.

---

78. a.F   b.F   c.T   d.F   e.T

Chemotherapy produces remission in around 80% of individuals.

Splenomegaly is not a common feature of AML. Thrombocytopenia, on the other hand, is a very frequent presentation.

Most people with AML are past retirement age.

Allogeneic BMT is the best form of cure but only one-third of individuals have a potential compatible sibling.

---

79. a.F   b.T   c.F   d.T   e.T

Folate deficiency causes macrocytic anaemia. β-Thalassaemia major and minor can cause microcytosis. Sickle cell disease is normocytic in nature. Rheumatoid arthritis can result in microcytosis due to iron deficiency as a result of NSAIDs or sometimes as a feature of the disease itself. Coeliac disease causes malabsorption of iron as well as folate.

---

80. a.T   b.F   c.F   d.T   e.F

Chronic joint disease is a very common feature of haemophilia A. Prior to factor VIII therapy, spontaneous cerebral haemorrhage was a common mode of death; HIV infection has overtaken this now.

The APTT is prolonged, not the prothrombin time. Fibrinogen levels are not affected. Gum bleeding is not a frequent feature of this disease.

---

81. a.T b.F c.F d.F e.T

Neutropenia is often a feature of acute leukaemia or follows a viral infection. Steroid therapy often produces a leucocytosis. Pregnancy often puts the neutrophil count up. Thalassaemia has no effect on the neutrophil count.

---

82. a.T b.F c.T d.T e.F

Activated protein C resistance (APCR) is the commonest form of inherited thrombophilia. It is due to factor V being resistant to activated protein C. This defect is present in about 5% of healthy controls and genetic analysis forms the best and most definitive means of diagnosis. It is equally common in both sexes.

---

83. a.T b.F c.F d.T e.T

People with coeliac disease undergo autosplenectomy. Patients with thalassaemia major often have splenomegaly and hypersplenism. Although autosplenectomy is a feature of sickle cell disease it is not a feature of sickle cell trait.

Amyloidosis and Gaucher's disease can infiltrate the spleen and cause a functional hyposplenism.

---

84. a.T b.F c.T d.T e.F

Phenytoin, septrin and chlorpromazine are all well recognized as causes of aplastic anaemia. Although interferon-α can reduce the neutrophil and platelet count it does not normally cause aplasia. Cimetidine does not normally affect the blood count.

---

85. a.T b.T c.T d.T e.T

Antilymphocyte globulin is raised in either rabbits or horses. It is produced by injecting human lymphocytes into these animals and harvesting the antihuman antibodies that are produced. It is quite effective in aplastic anaemia but has a number of side effects, some of which are quite severe due to the antigen–antibody reactions.

---

86. a.T b.T c.T d.F e.F

PNH can present with marrow hypoplasia, as can acute

lymphoblastic leukaemia. The inherited Fanconi's anaemia can present with aplasia or leukaemia.

Transfusion reactions do not result in hypoplasia.

The Blackfan–Diamond syndrome affects the red cell series only.

---

87. a.**T** b.**F** c.**T** d.**F** e.**T**

Chromosome 16 contains two active genes and two pseudo-genes (non-active) for α globin. Chromosome 11 possesses a single active gene with one pseudogene. Haemoglobin F is composed of two α and two γ chains. Haemoglobin H arises when no α chains can be produced, which results in the residual β chains forming a tetramer. Haemoglobin H runs very rapidly on haemoglobin electrophoresis (cellulose acetate).

---

88. a.**T** b.**F** c.**F** d.**T** e.**F**

Cold is a very common cause of crisis. These patients tend not to go bathing in the sea.

Even in the homozygous state a small amount of haemoglobin A may be formed.

The anaemia is normocytic. The haemoglobin S results from glutamic acid being substituted by valine at the six amino acid site of the β-globin gene.

The red cell lifespan is greatly reduced in sickle cell anaemia.

---

89. a.**F** b.**F** c.**T** d.**T** e.**T**

Immune haemolysis occurs in about 10% of patients with B-CLL.

Hyperleucocytosis is not usually a problem and may get into the 500 mark without any symptoms.

Classic phenotype of B-CLL is CD19 and 5 positive (this is unusual because the CD5 antigen is normally found on T cells).

Immunoglobulin levels are often reduced as part of the incompetent immune system. As a consequence of this immunosurveillance is deranged and monoclonal proteins can arise in up to 10% of cases.

90. a.T   b.F   c.T   d.T   e.T

Primary proliferative polycythaemia (PPP) replaces the old term polycythaemia rubra vera.

Plasma volume is usually normal although the red cell mass is always raised at diagnosis.

Venesection is the treatment of choice and suits most patients.

Splenomegaly is present in over 50% of patients.

It is a well-recognized feature that in PPP erythroid cells can grow in vitro without the support of erythropoietin. Marrow cells from normal individuals require erythropoietin to be added to the culture.

91. a.T   b.F   c.T   d.T   e.T

The majority of patients with β-thalassaemia major are treated with a blood transfusion regimen plus iron chelation. Transplantation is an option usually in children. Leg ulcers are more a feature of sickle cell anaemia than thalassaemia.

Pseudotumours can arise from soft tissues and are collections of extramedullary haemopoiesis. Microcytosis is a feature.

The predominant band on cellulose acetate is haemoglobin F which runs just behind the normal position of haemoglobin A.

92. a.F   b.T   c.T   d.T   e.F

There are many β-thalassaemia genetic abnormalities. The vast majority are point mutations rather than large gene deletions. In the heterozygous and homozygous states it confers a relative protection against malaria. The genetic mutation results in massive reduction or even absence of β-globin chain synthesis. Haemoglobin A2 is raised in β-thalassaemia trait but not in α-thalassaemia; it is also occasionally elevated in pernicious anaemia.

93. a.T   b.F   c.T   d.T   e.F

For children with severe anaemia and minimal liver fibrosis, transplantation is a good option. However, some patients with chronic iron overload will develop endocrinopathies which tend to be resistant to hormone replacement. Occasionally red cell transfusion requirements can be reduced by splenectomy. Although parenteral desferrioxamine is the standard treatment for iron chelation, oral agents are now becoming available. Blood transfusion regimens, if instituted early enough, can actually stop bone and soft tissue abnormalities developing.

---

94. a.**F** b.**F** c.**T** d.**F** e.**F**

LMW heparin does not cross the placenta and is not licensed in pregnancy. However, some pregnant women are treated with LMW heparin. Published data suggest that LMW heparin is superior as prophylaxis in orthopaedic surgery but not in general surgery. Unfractionated heparin has more antithrombin activity than LMW heparin.

---

95. a.**F** b.**F** c.**T** d.**T** e.**F**

HIT occurs in 1% of patients receiving unfractionated heparin. It is extremely rare with LMW heparin. New thromboembolic events are often seen in HIT and there is a high mortality of about 30%.

LMW crossreacts with unfractionated heparin, therefore it is better to use a heparinoid, e.g. danaparoid.

---

96. a.**T** b.**F** c.**T** d.**F** e.**F**

Vitamin K-dependent proteins involved in the coagulation system require carboxylation of their glutamic acids to become active. Warfarin inhibits vitamin K reductase and stops this carboxylation. The resulting proteins induced by vitamin K absence (PIVKA) have no clotting properties and can actually inhibit the action of remaining clotting factors.

Factor VII and protein C are amongst the first factors to fall following warfarin therapy; this can result in a prothrombotic tendency at day 1–2 of warfarin and heparinization should be adequate.

Breastfeeding is safe on warfarin.

---

97. a.**T** b.**T** c.**F** d.**F** e.**T**

NSAIDs are often protein bound and can therefore displace warfarin.

Tricyclics do suppress hepatic microenzyme activity.

Although phenytoin induces hepatic enzyme activity, this shortens the INR rather than prolonging it.

Antibiotics reduce the bacterial content of the gut and therefore reduce vitamin K production and absorption. Thyroxine modulates the hepatic receptor for warfarin.

---

98. a.**F** b.**F** c.**T** d.**F** e.**T**

Antithrombin III deficiency is inherited in an autosomal dominant manner. It accounts for less than 5% of recurrent thromboembolism. Because heparin has its action through antithrombin III, deficiency of ATIII will produce a relative heparin resistance. Prophylactic anticoagulation is indicated for all individuals in pregnancy and surgery but not for completely healthy individuals with no previous thromboembolic history.

---

99. a.**T** b.**F** c.**F** d.**T** e.**T**

ATIII deficiency causes more venous thrombosis than arterial thrombosis. The deficiency results from point mutations within the ATIII gene rather than gene deletion. ATIII deficiency is less common than protein C deficiency. It can manifest in the heterozygous form and may be due to abnormal function of the protein rather than a reduction in the quantity of the protein.

---

100. a.**F** b.**F** c.**T** d.**T** e.**T**

The homozygous form of protein C deficiency is devastating and is often fatal soon after birth. Heterozygous protein C deficiency commonly causes more venous than arterial thrombosis. Warfarinization can be hazardous because skin necrosis is a well-recognized feature in protein C-deficient patients receiving warfarin.

Protein C deficiency is dominantly inherited.

Protein C can be lost in the urine and this is why nephrotic syndrome is often associated with a thrombotic risk.

Infectious disease

101. Are the following statements about malaria seen in Britain true or false?

    a. The majority of cases occur in expatriates working overseas

    b. Malaria acquired in East and Central Africa is only caused by *Plasmodium falciparum* or *P. malariae*

    c. Malaria can be excluded by two negative thick blood films performed 12 h apart

    d. Patients who have acquired vivax malaria in the Indian subcontinent should be treated with quinine

    e. 'Radical cure' of vivax malaria with primaquine is unsuccessful in 10–15% of cases

102. Mefloquine chemoprophylaxis for malaria is characterized by:

    a. Side effects being more common in men

    b. Similar efficacy to the combination of chloroquine 300 mg weekly and proguanil 100 mg daily in preventing malaria in Africa

    c. A high incidence of drug-induced photosensitivity

    d. Severe side effects in 1/100 000 recipients

    e. Safety in pregnancy

103. Hydatid cystic disease is:

    a. Most likely to be localized in the lung

    b. Usually accompanied by peripheral eosinophilia

    c. Confirmed by examination of concentrated faecal specimens

    d. Usually parasitologically sterile if the cyst wall is heavily calcified

    e. Potentially treatable by elective cyst aspiration and instillation of hypertonic saline solution

104. Amoebic liver abscess is:

    a. Confirmed by the presence of *Entamoeba histolytica* cysts in faeces

    b. Ruled out by persistently negative amoebic serology

    c. Most common in the left lobe of the liver

    d. Typically associated with jaundice

    e. Treatable with chloroquine

105. Gastroenteritis caused by infection with *Escherichia coli* 0157 is:

    a. Always associated with blood in the faeces

    b. Usually diagnosed by faecal culture

    c. Associated with Henoch–Schönlein purpura

    d. Acquired from undercooked meat

    e. Best treated aggressively with antibiotics

106. Are the following statements concerning methicillin-resistant *Staphylococcus aureus* (MRSA) true or false?

    a. All carriers should be treated with mupirocin

    b. Colonization of a patient is usually followed by invasive infection

    c. Relatives of a carrier in the community should be screened for infection and treated

    d. The nationwide increase in infections is primarily due to the spread of the EMRSA-14 strain

    e. Invasive infection should be treated with third-generation cephalosporins

107. Are the following statements about infection with hepatitis C true or false?

    a. Approximately 25% of patients with positive anti-HCV antibodies will have no detectable virus by PCR tests

    b. The risk of sexual transmission from male to female is about 20%

    c. The risk of transmission from mother to fetus/infant in about 20%

    d. Hepatoma (hepatocellular carcinoma) complicates chronic infection in about 20% of cases

    e. Infection may be associated with autoimmune thyroid disease

108. The following infections are recognized complications of unscreened transfusion or sharing needles:

a. Chagas' disease
b. Malaria
c. Leishmaniasis
d. HTLV-II
e. Melioidosis

109. *Clostridium difficile* infection:

a. May be caused by metronidazole
b. May be treated with metronidazole
c. Can be prevented with vancomycin prophylaxis
d. Recurs in 50% of patients within 4 weeks
e. Is typically acquired from damp hospital fomites such as ventilator condensation traps, sinks, etc.

110. *Giardia lamblia* infection:

a. Is a typical zoonosis
b. Is common in patients with immunoglobulin deficiencies
c. Is typically more severe in patients with HIV infection
d. Is easily diagnosed by faecal culture
e. Is sometimes resistant to tinidazole in vitro

111. Microsporidial infection in man is:

a. Associated with travel to the tropics
b. Associated with conjunctivitis and sinusitis
c. Usually treatable with mebendazole
d. Prevented by prophylaxis with paromomycin
e. Diagnosed by staining faeces with photoreactive chemicals

112. Spongiform encephalopathy is:

a. Associated with abnormal carbohydrate fibrils in neuronal tissue
b. More common in individuals who are homozygous for HLA B27
c. Prevented by cooking infected meat thoroughly
d. Only found in Britain
e. Transmitted transplacentally in animals

113. Infection with schistosomiasis:

    a. Is often asymptomatic
    b. Can cause lumpy semen
    c. Is usually treated with oxamniquine injections
    d. Can cause wheezing, headache, fever and rash
    e. Is normally acquired by drinking contaminated water

114. In a patient presenting with fever after travel to India:

    a. Malaria can be excluded if the travel occurred more than 6 months previously
    b. Previous immunization against dengue rules out dengue fever
    c. The presence of diarrhoea rules out typhoid fever
    d. Regular malaria prophylaxis while abroad excludes malaria
    e. A platelet count of $120 \times 10^9/1$ suggests that malaria is the most likely diagnosis

115. A young woman presents with fever, headache, a stiff neck and a petechial rash. She has already received amoxycillin at home for 1 day:

    a. Microscopy of smears from the skin lesions may assist with the diagnosis
    b. The CSF cell count will already have returned to normal
    c. PCR testing of the CSF may help to confirm a diagnosis of meningococcal disease
    d. All family members should have throat swabs taken
    e. Family members should receive immediate meningococcal vaccination

116. Hepatitis E:

    a. Is more common in pregnant women
    b. Can cause lethal infection in neonates
    c. Produces solid immunity against reinfection
    d. Has an incubation period of 2–6 months
    e. Is restricted to the Indian subcontinent

117. In streptococcal infections:

    a. Erysipelas is characterized by necrosis of underlying muscle and fat

    b. Streptococcal glomerulonephritis is associated with pyoderma

    c. Erythema nodosum is a recognized sequel

    d. Treatment of uncomplicated streptococcal pharyngitis with a 5-day course of penicillin is sufficient to prevent rheumatic fever

    e. Necrotizing fasciitis is usually caused by group C streptococci

118. Are the following statements concerning urinary tract infection true or false?

    a. Recurrent urinary infection associated with staghorn calculi is usually due to pseudomonas infection

    b. Otherwise uncomplicated urinary tract infection in a young woman is best treated with a 5-day course of antibiotics

    c. Isolation of *Candida* spp. from a catheter specimen of urine should usually prompt treatment with systemic antifungals

    d. Microbiology laboratories use a different threshold for reporting antimicrobial resistance in bacterial isolates from urine, compared to isolates from other sites

    e. Young men should undergo full urological investigation after two proven urinary tract infections

119. These vectors transmit the following diseases:

    a. Tsetse flies and *Loa loa*

    b. Aedes mosquitoes and yellow fever

    c. Aedes mosquitoes and dengue fever

    d. Soft ticks and *Ehrlichia chafeensis*

    e. Hard ticks and *Borrelia burgdorferi*

120. The following infections may be transmitted to humans from cattle:

    a. Brucellosis

    b. Tuberculosis

    c. Leptospirosis

    d. Yersiniosis

    e. Orf

---

121. In a patient with falciparum malaria, the following are recognized indicators of severe infection:

    a. Platelet count below $90 \times 10^9/l$
    b. Parasitaemia >1%
    c. Convulsions
    d. Blood glucose less than 3 mmol/l
    e. Incubation period more than 7 days

---

122. For patients with tuberculosis:

    a. Active disease is excluded by a non-reactive tuberculin test
    b. Patients with coincident HIV infection need to be treated with two extra antituberculous drugs
    c. Patients with tuberculous meningitis should be nursed in an isolation cubicle
    d. Routine chemotherapy for pulmonary tuberculosis should continue for 9 months
    e. The chest X-ray may be negative in miliary disease

---

123. With regard to pneumococcal disease:

    a. Penicillin resistance is tested for by screening for in vitro resistance to penicillin discs
    b. The prevalence of multiresistant *S. pneumoniae* in the UK is <1%
    c. Multiresistant strains of *S. pneumoniae* are not prevented by the currently available vaccines
    d. Multiresistant pneumococcal infection can be treated with meropenem
    e. Steroids facilitate cefotaxime penetration into CSF to treat multiresistant pneumococcal meningitis

---

124. The following infections may be acquired by direct contact with soil/sand:

    a. Cutaneous larva migrans
    b. *Diphyllobothrium latum*
    c. *Necator americanus*
    d. *Ascaris lumbricoides*
    e. *Neospora caninum*

125. Which of the following statements concerning hepatitis B infection are true?

    a. Mutations of the surface antigen are associated with fulminant neonatal hepatitis

    b. A 20-year-old with acute symptomatic hepatitis B has a 10% chance of becoming a chronic carrier

    c. A chronic carrier with positive anti-HBe antibodies will not be infectious to others

    d. Lamivudine therapy is effective treatment for chronic carriage but there is rebound viraemia on discontinuation of therapy

    e. Most chronic carriers are female

126. Generalized seizures may be precipitated by treatment with:

    a. Benzylpenicillin

    b. Gentamicin

    c. Mefloquine

    d. Rifampicin

    e. Ciprofloxacin

127. There is a significant risk of intrauterine fetal damage after the following infections or immunizations:

    a. Herpes zoster (shingles)

    b. HIV

    c. Parvovirus B19

    d. Rubella vaccine

    e. Oral polio vaccine

128. In the diagnosis and management of infective endocarditis:

    a. At least six blood cultures are necessary for bacteriologic diagnosis

    b. Blood cultures yielding coagulase-negative staphylococci can be ignored unless the patient has a prosthetic heart valve

    c. Repeat echocardiography is mandatory for posttreatment monitoring

    d. For streptococcal infections, additional aminoglycoside therapy is essential if the MBC for penicillin is > 1 mg/l

    e. After streptococcal endocarditis prophylactic oral penicillin should be advised for at least 5 years

129. Varicella-zoster immune globulin (VZIG) is indicated for the prevention of chickenpox in:

    a. Pregnancy
    b. AIDS
    c. Asthmatics
    d. Neonates
    e. Common variable immunodeficiency

130. Adult bacterial gastroenteritis may be associated with:

    a. Erythema nodosum
    b. Urethritis
    c. Acute haemolysis
    d. Thrombocytosis
    e. Generalized seizures

131. Epstein–Barr virus (EBV) infection may cause:

    a. Severe thrombocytopenia
    b. Bullous myringitis
    c. Facial palsy
    d. Chronic persistent hepatitis
    e. Myocarditis

132. Jaundice may be a complication of treatment with:

    a. Flucloxacillin
    b. Nalidixic acid
    c. Cotrimoxazole
    d. Fusidic acid
    e. Coamoxyclav

133. In HIV-positive patients there is a link between:

    a. Human herpes virus type 8 and Kaposi's sarcoma
    b. Cytomegalovirus (CMV) and acalculous cholecystitis
    c. Epstein–Barr virus and primary intracranial lymphoma
    d. Papovavirus and rectal carcinoma
    e. Papillomavirus and oral hairy leucoplakia

134. Prognosis in HIV-associated *Pneumocystis carinii* pneumonia (PCP) is related to:

a. Extent of initial radiological involvement
b. Treatment with systemic corticosteroids
c. Degree of hypoxia on presentation
d. CD4 count
e. Presence of a preexisting AIDS-defining condition

135. The following factors decrease the likelihood of successful hepatitis B immunization:

a. Smoking
b. IV drug abuse
c. Age >40
d. Presence of serum antibody to hepatitis B core antigen
e. Asian origin

136. In the treatment of HIV infection the following drug combinations are associated with pharmacokinetic interactions:

a. Zidovudine and stavudine (d4T)
b. Lamivudine (3TC) and zalcitabine (ddC)
c. Ritonavir and cisapride
d. Saquinavir and grapefruit juice
e. Zidovudine and rifampicin .

137. Acute primary toxoplasmosis:

a. Is a hazard to the fetus only in the first two trimesters
b. May be transmitted by blood transfusion
c. May be diagnosed by PCR of peripheral blood
d. Is accompanied by peripheral blood eosinophilia
e. Accounts for 90% of cases of brain abscesses in AIDS

138. Corticosteroids are effective therapy in:

a. Tuberculous pericarditis
b. Guillain–Barré syndrome
c. Pyogenic meningitis in children
d. Herpes zoster
e. Glandular fever

139. The following may cause damage to peripheral nerves:

  a. HIV
  b. *Campylobacter jejuni*
  c. *Corynebacterium diphtheriae*
  d. Coxsackie viruses
  e. *Borrelia burgdorferi*

140. In HIV infection protease inhibitors:

  a. Have little effect on viral load when used as monotherapy
  b. Are rendered ineffective by rifampicin
  c. Are compatible with non-nucleoside reverse transcriptase inhibitors
  d. Prolong survival even in advanced disease
  e. Penetrate well into brain and CSF

141. Oesophagitis in AIDS may be caused by:

  a. Herpes simplex virus
  b. Cytomegalovirus
  c. *Cryptococcus neoformans*
  d. Epstein–Barr virus
  e. Kaposi's sarcoma

142. The following infections may cause uveitis:

  a. Shigella dysentery
  b. Herpes zoster
  c. Meningococcal septicaemia
  d. Loaiasis
  e. Enterovirus 70

143. The following are indications for pneumococcal vaccination:

  a. Coeliac disease
  b. Sickle cell trait
  c. Alcoholic cirrhosis
  d. HIV infection
  e. Recurrent frontal sinusitis

144. In human rabies:

  a. There is no history of an animal bite in 20% of cases

b. Skin biopsies are helpful in diagnosis
c. There is a significant risk of infection spreading to intensive care staff nursing the patient
d. The incubation period is significantly longer in children
e. There is no hazard to man from birds or reptiles

145. In gonococcal arthropathy:

a. The organism is nearly always resistant to penicillin
b. 60% of patients will have symptoms of urethritis
c. Skin lesions resemble those found in meningococcal septicaemia and contain immune complexes
d. The gonococcal complement fixation test is used to confirm the diagnosis
e. Joint fluid is invariably sterile on culture

146. Parvovirus B19 infection causes:

a. An acute fall in haemoglobin in previously healthy individuals
b. Erythema subitum
c. Hydrops fetalis
d. Chronic encephalopathy in advanced AIDS
e. Chronic viraemia lasting a year or longer

147. In Weil's disease (leptospirosis):

a. The platelet count is usually normal
b. Blood cultures are most likely to be positive during the second week of illness
c. Penicillin therapy improves renal function
d. Treatment must include measures to prevent hepatic encephalopathy
e. Elevated creatine kinase levels are common

148. Acute adrenal failure may complicate:

a. Tuberculosis
b. Cytomegalovirus infection
c. Meningococcal septicaemia
d. Histoplasmosis
e. Staphylococcal toxic shock

149. In Lassa fever:

    a. The patient's body fluids are a major crossinfection hazard during the incubation period

    b. The polymerase chain reaction (PCR) is used for early diagnosis

    c. The disease has an insidious onset with haemorrhage occurring late

    d. Antiviral therapy is ineffective

    e. Mortality is higher in primary than in secondary cases

150. Fluoroquinolone antibiotics:

    a. Are useful in the treatment of *Mycobacterium avium* infection in AIDS

    b. Reduce the duration of salmonella enteritis by at least 5 days

    c. Reach high levels in CSF

    d. Are associated with Achilles tendon rupture

    e. Act by inhibiting bacterial DNA gyrase

101. a.F b.F c.F d.F e.T

The largest epidemiological group (about 50%) importing malaria infection to Britain includes people visiting friends and relatives who live in malaria-endemic regions. Holidaymakers and expatriates working overseas account for approximately 20% and 5% of imported cases respectively. While most malaria acquired in East/Central Africa is likely to be caused by *Plasmodium falciparum*, about 5–10% of cases are caused by *P. vivax*.

In a patient with possible malaria, two negative blood films only 12 h apart are insufficient to exclude the diagnosis, particularly if parasitaemia has been partially suppressed by chemoprophylaxis or empirical treatment. Further films will need to be performed, possibly supplemented by antigen detection tests such as the 'Parasight F' or the 'ICT'.

Vivax malaria almost invariably responds to chloroquine which remains the first-line treatment of choice, although chloroquine-resistant strains have been reported in Oceania and in the Indian subcontinent. However, quinine can be used to treat vivax malaria and might be indicated if there was uncertainty about species identification and the possibility of falciparum malaria had not been ruled out. Primaquine therapy is required to prevent recrudescence of vivax malaria arising from hypnozoites in the liver; it has long been known that the Chesson strain of vivax prevalent in Papua New Guinea, Irian Jaya and the Solomons is relatively resistant to primaquine. More recently, failure rates of about 10–15% have been reported with vivax acquired elsewhere.

102. a.F b.F c.F d.F e.F

Side effects of mefloquine are more frequently reported by women than by men, but do not include photosensitivity, which is more commonly associated with doxycycline chemoprophylaxis. The incidence of severe side effects reported in surveillance studies varies, but is of the order of one in 10 000 recipients, not one in 100 000. The protective efficacy of mefloquine in Africa is superior to the usual recommended prophylactic regimen of chloroquine two tablets (300 mg) weekly and proguanil two tablets (200 mg) daily and is certainly more effective than the inadequate comparative regimen containing only one tablet (100 mg) of proguanil a day. Until recently, pregnancy or the possibility of becoming pregnant was thought to be an absolute contraindication to mefloquine therapy, but surveillance of women who have inadvertently become pregnant while taking mefloquine has failed to show any excess fetal problems. Many authorities would still recommend an alternative regimen for women known to be pregnant.

---

103. a.**F**   b.**F**   c.**F**   d.**T**   e.**T**

Hydatid disease, due to the presence of tissue cysts of the dog tapeworm *Echinococcus granulosus*, is most commonly localized in the liver (about 70% of cases). The lung is the next most common site, in about 15% of cases.

Although peripheral eosinophilia is seen in many helmintic infections it is only found in about 10% of hydatid cases and when present may indicate cyst leakage or rupture. Hydatid material (usually hooklets from the protoscolices) is only found in human faeces after rupture of cyst contents down the biliary tree into the gastrointestinal tract. The adult worm does not colonize human gut.

Cysts with heavily calcified walls have been present for many years and are usually (but not always) parasitologically sterile. Such cysts do not usually need therapeutic intervention unless a complication has occurred such as bacterial superinfection, traumatic rupture or local pressure effects. Solitary uncalcified cysts in the liver may respond to chemotherapy with agents such as albendazole and/or praziquantel, although resective surgery will often be needed as well. Several series have now demonstrated the feasibility and safety of treatment by aspiration, percutaneous instillation of a scolicidal agent such as hypertonic saline and reaspiration of cyst contents via a wide-bore catheter. Such treatment is only currently used under carefully controlled conditions in centres with considerable experience.

---

104. a.**F**   b.**T**   c.**F**   d.**F**   e.**T**

The presence or absence of amoebic cysts or trophozoites in faeces has no useful predictive value in the diagnosis of amoebic liver abscess and there may or may not be a history of associated diarrhoea. Jaundice is rare and the diagnosis is usually suggested by clinical features, peripheral neutrophilia and imaging findings including a raised right hemidiaphragm with or without reactive changes in the right lung base and sonographic or CT evidence of abscess. Serological tests are usually positive at clinical presentation, but may rarely be negative in the initial stages of illness and the test should be repeated if clinical suspicion continues. The majority of solitary abscesses are in the right lobe of the liver. Cysts in the left lobe have a higher associated morbidity, including the possibility of rupture into the pericardium, and location in the left lobe is a relative indication for elective therapeutic aspiration of cyst content. The usual treatment is with metronidazole or tinidazole, but chloroquine is also effective against liver abscesses.

---

105. a.F b.F c.F d.T e.F

Although bloody diarrhoea is one of the typical features of *E. coli* 0157 infection, there may be little diarrhoea and blood may be absent. Diagnosis is usually made by screening for the presence of enterohaemorrhagic toxin in faeces, although faecal culture and identification of the strains by agglutination tests is an adjunctive investigation. One of the major complications of *E. coli* 0157 infection is haemolytic uraemic syndrome (HUS), particularly in young boys and the elderly.

Sources of infection include uncooked meats, cooked meat contaminated by organisms transferred from uncooked meat, and milk.

Observational studies suggest that aggressive and early antibiotic treatment may be implicated in precipitating HUS and many practitioners would withhold antibiotics for this reason. However, there are no controlled prospective studies to confirm this clinical observation.

---

106. a.F b.F c.F d.F e.F

Many patients are colonized without developing invasive infection. The role of treatments such as topical mupirocin to clear nasal colonization remains controversial, even for hospitalized patients, and the evidence base for its use in hospital staff who are carriers is also poor. Such treatment is unlikely to be advised for carriers who are living in the general community. Similarly, the main risk a carrier poses is to other debilitated patients in a hospital or nursing home situation and family members are not usually regarded as being at risk unless they have severe multisystem disease.

The widespread increase in MRSA infection throughout health-care institutions in Britain is due to several different strains of MRSA, including EMRSA-3, -15 and -16 but not typically EMRSA-14. The major problem for patients is invasive infection, which is often resistant to cephalosporin treatment. First-line treatment usually includes vancomycin or, in some institutions, teicoplanin. The emergence of vancomycin-resistant strains of MRSA is not yet a major numerical problem in Britain but will require novel antibiotic approaches.

---

107. a.**T**   b.**F**   c.**F**   d.**F**   e.**T**

The majority of patients infected by hepatitis C become chronic carriers, as evidenced by positive PCR tests for serum RNA. In some patients whose serum PCR tests are negative, HCV RNA can still be detected in liver tissue.

The risk of sexual transmission is generally lower than 5% for long-term female partners of infected males. The risk is reduced considerably if the male is consistently PCR negative. Maternal transmission of infection is of the order of 5–10% in most series and again is markedly lower if the mother is HCV PCR negative. However, the majority of infants born to antibody-positive mothers will have positive antibody tests for several months after delivery due to transplacental transfer of maternal antibody. This does not indicate active infection of the infant, which can only be ruled out by extended follow-up for loss of maternal antibody and/or persistently negative PCR tests.

The natural history of chronic hepatitis C varies with the route of infection and viral inoculum and appears to be more benign after a single exposure to low viral load. Follow-up of heavily infected patients (after transfusion of infected blood) suggests that about 20–50% will eventually develop cirrhosis; thereafter the risk of hepatocellular carcinoma is about 3–5% per year, although this risk is increased if the patient abuses alcohol.

Hepatitis C infection may be associated with a variety of abnormal immune phenomena including cryoglobulinaemia and autoimmune thyroid disease. Thyroid disease may be exacerbated by interferon therapy.

108. a.T b.T c.T d.T e.T

Chagas' disease (*Trypanosoma cruzi*) in South and Central America may be an asymptomatic infection for many years and poses a genuine transfusion hazard. Patients who have lived in endemic areas should be excluded from blood donation unless their blood has been screened.

Malaria (caused by any species) is a potential transfusion hazard for several years after the donor has left a malarious area. Malaria transmission via blood stored for months has also been documented. Immune screening tests for malaria in blood donations in the UK are currently being evaluated.

Leishmaniasis is recognized to be a transfusion hazard. There is reasonable epidemiological evidence to suggest that much of the visceral leishmaniasis seen in HIV-positive Spanish IV drug misusers is due to needle sharing.

All retroviruses may be transmitted by transfusion and/or needle sharing; HTLV-II is not as common in risk groups in the UK as in the USA and the screening of blood donors in the UK for this infection is still under debate.

Melioidosis, caused by the soil-associated organism *Burkholderia pseudomallei*, can be transmitted by transfusion as well as by direct inoculation and was first described in morphine addicts in Burma.

109. a.T b.T c.F d.F e.F

Metronidazole is one of the many antibiotics that has been implicated in triggering *Cl. difficile* infection and can also be used to treat it with similar efficacy to vancomycin. Primary prophylaxis with vancomycin is not effective for prevention of a first attack of *Cl. difficile* diarrhoea. Although many patients continue to excrete spores in faeces after treatment and up to 25% have further clinical illness within 4 weeks, secondary prophylaxis with vancomycin does not prevent this either.

Cl. difficile is difficult to eradicate from dry ward surfaces. Moist areas such as condensation traps are more typically associated with nosocomial infection with Gram-negative organisms such as *Pseudomonas* spp., Serratia, etc.

110. a.F b.T c.F d.F e.T

There are several species of giardia, some associated with

specific animal hosts. Although some infections of humans have been associated with mammals, e.g. waterborne outbreaks related to beavers, most human infections are not zoonotic. Immunoglobulin deficiency syndromes are often associated with giardiasis which may be difficult to eradicate and patients with persistent giardiasis should be screened for serum immunoglobulin deficiency.

Patients with HIV may be at more risk of acquiring *G. lamblia* due to their lifestyle, but such infections are not generally more severe clinically than in HIV-negative individuals, although they may be more persistent. Diagnosis is usually confirmed by faecal microscopy or antigen detection, although occasionally upper intestinal fluid or biopsy may need to be examined. Culture of faeces is feasible but is not routinely employed for diagnosis and axenic cultures of *G. lamblia* may show resistance to metronidazole or tinidazole. The clinical significance of such resistance remains uncertain.

---

111. a.**T**   b.**T**   c.**F**   d.**F**   e.**T**

As serological techniques for diagnosis have become available, the widespread prevalence of microsporidial infection in the tropics has become apparent. Travellers to the tropics have more serological evidence of infection than non-travellers, irrespective of any immunodeficiency. Several genera of microsporidia are associated with infection of the respiratory tract and/or eyes, sometimes with dissemination to other sites, particularly in patients with AIDS.

Infections with *Encephalitozoon* spp. sometimes respond to albendazole (not mebendazole) therapy, but the most common microsporidial cause of diarrhoea in AIDS patients, *Enterocytozoon bieneusi*, is less likely to respond. Paromomycin is a non-absorbable aminoglycoside used with limited effect in the treatment of cryptosporidiosis complicating HIV infection. It has no role in the prevention or treatment of microsporidial infection. The laboratory investigation of microsporidial diarrhoea is time-consuming and the spores are difficult to visualize using conventional stains. Transmission electron microscopy of small bowel biopsy remains the gold standard, but stool microscopy after modified trichrome staining or fluorescence microscopy of faeces stained with chromotropic stains such as Uvitex B or calcofluor may facilitate diagnosis. PCR-based techniques may supplement or replace these techniques as they are improved upon in the future.

---

112. a.F   b.F   c.F   d.F   e.T

The spongiform encephalopathies are associated with abnormal prion proteins in the brain and human disease may be inherited, acquired or sporadic. The rarer inherited forms of Creutzfeldt–Jakob disease (CJD) and similar human spongiform encephalopathies are autosomal dominant disorders associated with coding mutations in the prion protein gene. Most sporadic cases of human spongiform encephalopathy are not due to CJD but to 'new variant CJD', which has characteristically different neuropathological appearances and may be the human counterpart of bovine spongiform encephalopathy (BSE). The infective agent is heat resistant and can survive temperatures far higher than those obtained during routine cooking of meat. BSE has been reported in several European countries both in cattle and in man. As with most spongiform encephalopathies, it is transmitted transplacentally.

---

113. a.T   b.T   c.F   d.T   e.F

Infection is frequently asymptomatic. Infection of the male genitourinary tract can result in a number of symptoms including haematuria, discoloration of semen and 'lumpy' semen and occasionally frank haematospermia. In the past oxamniquine was the mainstay of treatment for *S. mansoni* infections, but praziquantel is now regarded as first-line chemotherapy for all species. The symptoms of acute schistosomal infection are only reported by newly exposed patients – so-called 'Katayama fever'. These are allergic reactions to migrating schistosomules and typically include headache, wheezing, transient urticarial rashes, cough, fever and eosinophilia.

Schistosomiasis is usually contracted by contact of skin with infected fresh water, followed by invasion of the skin by schistosomal cercariae. It is theoretically possible for cercariae to penetrate buccal mucosa if infected water is taken by mouth and potentially infective water should be filtered and allowed to stand for 48 h before being drunk if chlorination is not possible.

114. a.F   b.F   c.F   d.F   e.F

Almost all patients with falciparum malaria present within 2 months of leaving a malarious area, but vivax infections are frequently seen 6–12 months or longer after trips to the Indian subcontinent.

No vaccine is available against dengue fever, although vaccination against Japanese encephalitis may provide some protection against dengue.

Diarrhoea is often a feature of acute falciparum malaria, but is also seen in typhoid or paratyphoid fever, especially in children.

Adherence to regular malaria chemoprophylaxis does not provide complete protection – the regimen may be inappropriate for the area, the traveller may not fully comply with the regimen or there may have been poor absorption of drugs due to gastrointestinal illness. Inadequate prophylaxis may prolong the incubation period and often slows the progression of clinical disease so that patients have longer in which to seek medical attention.

Patients with acute malaria often have mild thrombocytopenia which is usually more severe with falciparum malaria. The important imported fevers in the differential diagnosis (arboviruses, enteric fever, rickettsial infections) also produce mild thrombocytopenia so a platelet count of this level does not have strong specific diagnostic value but should still prompt a careful search for malaria parasites. Conversely, a normal platelet count (approximately 25% of acute malaria cases) does not have useful negative predictive value.

115. a.T   b.F   c.T   d.F   e.F

In expert hands, smears taken from the skin rash caused by meningococcal disease can be stained with Gram's or Giemsa stains to show diplococci and sometimes yield positive cultures despite negative blood cultures.

It takes at least several days for the cerebrospinal fluid white count and biochemistry to return to normal after effective treatment for bacterial meningitis, although the cell pattern may not be so 'typical' of pyogenic meningitis during the recovery phase. In practice, this means that lumbar puncture can be delayed and performed later if still needed for diagnostic purposes, while treatment is initiated without delay. The recent introduction of PCR-based tests for use in both CSF and peripheral blood has been a clinically useful advance in the diagnosis of culture-negative meningococcal meningitis, particularly in situations like this where the patient has already received antibiotics.

Family members and 'kissing contacts' of the patient should receive immediate chemoprophylaxis with rifampicin or ciprofloxacin, but there is no evidence that taking routine throat swabs is of any benefit as it does not influence the management decision to institute prophylaxis. It is not yet routine practice to offer immediate vaccination to family members except in an epidemic caused by a known strain because the majority of sporadic British cases of meningococcal disease are caused by group B strains for which there is no vaccine. However, the family may subsequently be offered vaccination if the index case is shown to be infected with a group A or C strain, against which there are effective vaccines.

---

116. a.**F**   b.**T**   c.**F**   d.**F**   e.**F**

Hepatitis E causes severe hepatitis in pregnant women and transplacental/perinatal spread with high neonatal mortality rates have now been recognized too. However, there is no evidence that infection is more frequent in pregnant than in other women.

Infection does not appear to induce prolonged solid immunity; evidence for this includes infections of young adults in apparent endemic areas and the failure of immune globulin, derived from adults in endemic areas, to protect against infection. The incubation period is about 2–6 weeks and infection is widespread in the tropics, including North and East Africa and Central and South America, in addition to the regions surrounding the Indian subcontinent.

---

117. a.**F**   b.**T**   c.**T**   d.**F**   e.**F**

Erysipelas is a distinct clinical form of cellulitis characterized by sharply demarcated margins of rash and involvement of subcutaneous tissue. Necrosis of underlying muscle and fat is a feature of necrotizing fasciitis. The association of glomerulonephritis as a sequel of streptococcal skin infection is well characterized, whereas rheumatic fever is typically a sequel of pharyngeal infection.

Streptococcal infection is a common cause of erythema nodosum. While treatment of streptococcal pharyngitis with a

5-day course of penicillin may be adequate for control of local symptoms, it has long been recognized that a 10-day course of treatment is required in order to reduce the subsequent risk of developing rheumatic fever.

Necrotizing fasciitis, which has increased in incidence in many Western countries, is usually caused by group A streptococcal infection (*S. pyogenes*).

---

118. a.**F**   b.**F**   c.**F**   d.**T**   e.**T**

Staghorn calculi are more typically associated with *Proteus* spp. infections, characterized by urease production which raises urinary pH, promoting struvite stone formation.

Five days treatment would not be necessary for treatment of an uncomplicated urinary tract infection (UTI) in a young woman, which can often be treated with a single dose of antibiotic, and the course should certainly not exceed 3 days.

Colonization of urinary catheters with *Candida* spp. is a common occurrence and does not automatically indicate significant lower or higher UTI.

Coexisting factors suggesting significant candida infection would include lumbar and/or renal pain with fever, rigors and other features of dissemination, including candidaemia with or without IV lines and cutaneous lesions compatible with systemic disease.

Many antibiotics are concentrated in urine, so that the achievable levels usually greatly exceed the concentration needed to kill microorganisms. Thus, an organism that is only moderately sensitive in vitro may well respond in vivo. Many laboratories take this into account when reporting on urinary isolates of bacteria.

Young men who have repeated attacks of urinary tract infection should be fully investigated for underlying structural and other predisposing conditions, in addition to careful questioning about sexual practices and exclusion of sexually transmitted infections.

---

119. a.**F**   b.**T**   c.**T**   d.**F**   e.**T**

Tsetse flies transmit African trypanosomiasis, while *Loa loa* is transmitted by the bite of deer flies (*Chrysops* spp.). Urban spread of yellow fever virus (human–human) is usually mediated by *Aedes aegypti* while the sylvatic cycle (monkey–human) involves *Aedes* spp. or *Haemagogus* spp. Dengue fever is also typically spread by the bite of *Aedes aegypti*.

Most tickborne diseases that affect humans are transmitted by hard ticks, with the exception of endemic relapsing fever (*Borrelia duttoni*) which is transmitted by the soft tick *Ornithodorus moubata*. Ehrlichiosis is transmitted by hard ticks such as *Dermacentor variabilis* and *Amblyomma americanum*.

Lyme disease (*B. burgdorferi*) is a zoonosis that man acquires in saliva from the bite of hard ticks of the genus Ixodes, particularly *I. scapularis*.

---

120. a.**T** b.**T** c.**T** d.**T** e.**F**

Bovines (cattle, buffalo, bison, etc.) are naturally infected with *Brucella* spp., usually but not exclusively *B. abortus*, which is the archetypal zoonotic infection. Other animal hosts for *Brucella* include sheep, goats, camels and pigs. Control of human infection is achieved by public health and veterinary measures including immunization of animals, selective slaughter of infected herds and pasteurization of milk. Pasteurization and culling of infected animals are also used to control transmission of *Mycobacterium bovis* from cattle to man.

The different species of leptospira are typically associated with different animal vectors and situations. Milk-parlour and other dairy workers are at risk of acquiring *L. hardjo* which is excreted in cow's urine. Yersinia infections (*Y. tuberculosis* and *Y. pseudotuberculosis*) are more usually associated with animals such as deer or pigs but a wide variety of other animal hosts include cattle, while plague (*Y. pestis*) is associated with rats.

Orf is caused by a poxvirus that is acquired by direct contact with sheep and goats, which are often affected by lesions around the mouth.

---

121. a.**F** b.**F** c.**T** d.**T** e.**F**

Thrombocytopenia of this degree is common in malaria and is not an indicator of severe disease. A platelet count <20 000 would cause more concern, but is not a specific indicator of severity of infection.

In the context of a semiimmune patient in the tropics, the WHO definition of severe parasitaemia is >4%. In the British context of a non-immune patient with imported disease, most clinicians would regard a parasite rate of >2% as an indication for more aggressive chemotherapy.

Convulsions, which may be due to hypoglycaemia, fever or the malarial disease process itself, are an indicator of more severe disease, as is hypoglycaemia, risk factors for which include high parasitaemia, pregnancy and quinine therapy. The duration of the incubation period does not affect the severity of illness.

---

122. a.F b.F c.F d.F e.T

The tuberculin skin test represents a complex host reaction and may be falsely negative in many situations, including defects of host immunity (old age, HIV, etc.), poor-quality PPD, poor injecting technique and overwhelming tuberculous infection.

While patients with HIV are at increased risk of acquiring TB, they should respond to conventional therapy without additional concurrent antituberculous medication. However, the role and possible duration of extended treatment remain uncertain.

Patients with tuberculous meningitis do not need prolonged isolation, but their urine and/or sputum may be infectious to others if they have untreated miliary disease. These secretions (and CSF) should be rendered sterile within a few days of starting effective chemotherapy including rifampicin and isolation will not need to exceed 14 days.

British and many other national guidelines for treatment of uncomplicated pulmonary TB are for 6 months total treatment, with more intensive combinations during the first 2 months. The classic miliary pattern of shadowing may take some time to develop; the clinical relevance is that a patient with a PUO, who is suspected of having miliary TB, may need repeated chest X-rays to detect this.

---

123. a.F b.F c.F d.T e.F

Penicillin disc testing alone is technically inadequate and laboratories that use disc testing to screen usually use oxacillin discs as a more robust indicator of penicillin resistance.

Pneumococci that are at least partially resistant to penicillin now account for >4% of British isolates and the majority of these are also resistant to erythromycin and to other first-line antibiotics. While some capsular strains of pneumococci are more likely to be associated with resistance to antibiotics, these are usually preventable with commercially available vaccines. Multiresistant pneumococci may still be sensitive to agents such as vancomycin or cefotaxime. Meropenem has recently been shown to be a safe and viable alternative, particularly if there is resistance to the latter agents. Concurrent treatment of meningitis with cefotaxime and steroids leads to reduced CSF penetration of antibiotic and has been linked to therapeutic failures.

---

124. a.**T**   b.**F**   c.**T**   d.**F**   e.**F**

Cutaneous larva migrans is caused by localized skin infection by the larvae of cat or dog hookworms, acquired by lying, sitting or standing on sand or soil contaminated with animal faeces.

Diphyllobothrium latum is the fish tapeworm, the infective source of which is usually eating uncooked fish.

Hookworms (*Necator americanus* and *Ancylostoma duodenale*) have a lifecycle that includes ova being passed in human faeces onto the ground, where they mature and hatch to produce larval stages which can infect man by direct penetration of skin. In contrast, roundworms (*Ascaris lumbricoides*) are usually acquired by the faeco-oral route: very hardy eggs are excreted in human faeces and these hatch in the stomach of the next human to eat food contaminated by faeces.

Neospora caninum is a coccidian parasite of animals that is of uncertain significance as a zoonosis as transmission to humans has not yet been reported.

---

125. a.**F**   b.**F**   c.**F**   d.**T**   e.**F**

While mutations of HBsAg are recognized to be a cause for failure of vaccination, they are not usually associated with more fulminant disease: this is a feature of 'precore' mutations that lead to defective HBeAg production and is known to be associated with severe disease in neonates born to infected mothers.

Young adults who acquire hepatitis B are less likely to become carriers than neonates and infants and this progression to carriage is even less likely if the immune response is vigorous enough to produce symptoms. The risk is less than 5% and women are more likely to clear the infection than men, so the majority of chronic carriers are male.

The presence of anti-HBe antibody is a marker of relatively reduced viraemia and severity of liver disease, but carriers with anti-HBe are still infectious to others, especially the minority who have mutations of HBeAg.

Lamivudine is a nucleoside reverse transcriptase inhibitor currently undergoing trials in chronic hepatitis B and also in combinations of anti-HIV treatments. Suppression of HBV viraemia occurs rapidly, but is only sustained during treatment, with rebound viraemia after cessation of monotherapy. The role of lamivudine in combination with other antiviral therapy for HBV is still being explored.

---

126. a.**T** b.**F** c.**T** d.**F** e.**T**

Penicillins may produce encephalopathy, including fits, if given in large doses intravenously. Encephalopathy is more likely if the blood–brain barrier is impaired, e.g. by renal failure. Historically encephalopathy has also been described after intrathecal administration of excessive doses of benzylpenicillin.

Gentamicin penetrates poorly into CSF and brain. Its use is not associated with adverse CNS reactions, although it is of course ototoxic.

Neuropsychiatric symptoms and fits occur during malaria prophylaxis with mefloquine at a rate of approximately one in 10 000. A higher incidence is reported during treatment when larger doses are used. Patients with a history of psychiatric disturbances or convulsions should not be given mefloquine prophylactically.

Rifampicin does not itself cause fits. However, it reduces plasma levels of phenytoin by enzyme induction; epileptic patients receiving both drugs must therefore have their phenytoin levels monitored.

Ciprofloxacin should be used with caution in patients with epilepsy or CNS disorder as there is a risk of drug-induced fits. The risk is enhanced by coadministration with theophylline since plasma levels of theophylline are thereby increased.

---

127. a.**F** b.**F** c.**T** d.**F** e.**F**

Maternal herpes zoster (shingles) is not a risk to the fetus; on the other hand, chickenpox in the first trimester carries an approximately 1% risk of fetal damage.

In Europe about 14% of babies born to HIV-positive mothers will acquire HIV infection either in utero or peripartum. However, the virus does not appear to be teratogenic and there is no excess fetal loss.

Maternal parvovirus B19 infection does cause a small excess fetal loss, from anaemia and hydrops fetalis, especially during the second trimester.

There is evidence to suggest that rubella and polio vaccines are not teratogenic. Nevertheless, live vaccines should not be administered to pregnant women. Where there is a significant risk of exposure to the disease (e.g. poliomyelitis, yellow fever) the need for immunization outweighs any theoretical risk to the fetus.

---

128. a.F b.F c.F d.T e.F

Of patients with infective endocarditis in whom a bacterial diagnosis is eventually made, 95% can be successfully diagnosed by three blood cultures; additional cultures are only necessary to assess the significance of low virulence organisms such as coagulase-negative staphylococci. The latter can cause native valve endocarditis often in association with preexisting mitral valve prolapse: their significance should always be carefully considered, particularly if they are grown from multiple cultures.

Although echocardiography is useful in assessing valve function during active endocarditis, it is of little help during follow-up after treatment. At this stage monitoring is best carried out by recording clinical features, body temperature and results of peripheral white cell count and acute inflammatory markers.

For endocarditis caused by streptococci of reduced penicillin sensitivity (minimum bactericidal titre >1 mg/l), an aminoglycoside should be added to high-dose penicillin therapy for up to 4 weeks of treatment. Aminoglycoside blood levels should be carefully monitored.

Long-term prophylactic penicillin is indicated after rheumatic fever but has no role in the prevention of endocarditis.

---

129. a.T b.T c.F d.T e.F

Pregnant women in contact with chickenpox or herpes zoster, who do not have a previous history of varicella-zoster virus (VZV) infection, should have blood taken for VZV antibody testing. A rapid immunofluorescent method is available. Those lacking antibody should be given VZIG which attenuates maternal chickenpox; it may also provide some protection against fetal infection.

Patients with symptomatic HIV infection should be treated similarly; those without a previous VZV history should be screened serologically and given VZIG if seronegative. Asthmatics do not require VZIG unless they are receiving large doses of systemic corticosteroids.

VZIG is recommended for neonates at risk, up to 4 weeks after birth. Firstly, for those whose mothers develop chickenpox in the period 7 days to 1 month after delivery. Secondly, for those in contact with chickenpox or herpes zoster whose mothers have no history of chickenpox or who on testing have no antibody. Thirdly, for those in contact with chickenpox who are born before 30 weeks of gestation or with a birth weight of <1 kg. Patients with common variable immunodeficiency (agammaglobulinaemia) are not at risk from severe VZV if they are receiving immunoglobulin treatment.

---

130. a.**T**   b.**T**   c.**T**   d.**T**   e.**T**

Invasive bacterial gut pathogens (salmonellae, shigellae, campylobacter, *Yersinia* spp.) may cause erythema nodosum, with or without polyarthritis. Postdysenteric Reiter's syndrome, sometimes accompanied with conjunctivitis, uveitis and/or urethritis, may follow infection with the same group of organisms. The syndrome is linked to the HLA B27 phenotype.

E. coli 0157 produces cytotoxins which are responsible for the haemolytic – uraemic syndrome.

Thrombocytosis is usually suggestive of inflammatory bowel disease rather than gut infection unless the latter is accompanied by arthropathy, but is also seen during the late recovery phase after bacterial gastroenteritis.

Generalized seizures are uncommon during gastroenteritis in adults but are well recognized in association with shigella dysentery and campylobacter infection.

---

131. a.**T**   b.**F**   c.**T**   d.**F**   e.**T**

Severe thrombocytopenia is an unusual complication of infectious mononucleosis (IM) which may respond to corticosteroid therapy. Bullous myringitis does not occur in IM; it is a characteristic feature of *Mycoplasma pneumoniae* upper respiratory tract infection. Both polyneuritis and mononeuritis are well-recognized features of acute EBV infection with or without accompanying IM. Mononeuritis often manifests as facial palsy. Eighty percent of patients with IM will have abnormal liver function tests but histological liver damage is minimal and chronic liver disease has not been described. Transient ECG repolarization abnormalities are common in IM but are seldom clinically significant; symptomatic myocarditis is rare.

---

132. a.T b.T c.T d.T e.T

Jaundice can be an unusual unwanted effect of treatment with all the antimicrobials listed. Flucloxacillin and the clavulanic acid component of coamoxyclav are occasionally associated with hepatitis or cholestasis and high-dose treatment with flucloxacillin and other penicillins may induce antibody-mediated haemolysis. Reversible hepatic damage with jaundice may occur after oral or parenteral fusidic acid therapy. The sulphonamide component of cotrimoxazole, like other sulphonamides, can cause reversible chronic active hepatitis or induce haemolysis (especially in subjects deficient in erythrocyte glucose-6-phosphate dehydrogenase).

Kernicterus in the fetus is a potential hazard of sulphonamide therapy in pregnancy as these agents displace maternal protein-bound bilirubin.

Nalidixic acid does not cause liver damage but a variety of drug-induced haemolytic anaemias have been described after its use.

---

133. a.T b.T c.T d.F e.F

Almost all specimens of AIDS-associated Kaposi's sarcoma (KS) contain the DNA of human herpes virus type 8 (HHV8) and 75% of AIDS patients who have had KS for more than 5 years have PCR evidence of HHV8 in blood.

CMV infection in AIDS may produce vasculitic inflammation in the biliary tract, causing painful cholecystitis.

Rectal carcinoma prevalence is increased 100-fold in patients with HIV infection and is associated with papilloma virus infection of rectal mucosa.

A papovavirus (JC virus) is responsible for progressive multifocal leucoencephalopathy in AIDS. Oral hairy leucoplakia is related to Epstein–Barr virus (EBV) infection of the tongue epithelium and can be controlled with antivirals such as aciclovir. EBV is also associated with primary intracranial lymphoma in AIDS.

---

134. a.**F**   b.**T**   c.**T**   d.**T**   e.**F**

The extent of initial radiological involvement in PCP correlates poorly with severity or outcome. Hypoxia (arterial pO_2 <10 kPa on 35% oxygen) is a marker of poor prognosis, but mortality in this group of patients is reduced by treatment with corticosteroids. Mortality in PCP is increased in patients with CD4 counts of <50×10^6/L but is otherwise unaffected by the presence of a preexisting AIDS diagnosis.

---

135. a.**T**   b.**F**   c.**T**   d.**T**   e.**F**

Individuals aged over 40 years and those who smoke cigarettes are less likely to develop protective antibody after primary hepatitis B immunization. A history of intravenous drug abuse or Asian origin is irrelevant unless the subject has past or current hepatitis B infection. Vaccinees seropositive for hepatitis B core antibody (anti-HBc) will not respond to the vaccine.

---

136. a.**T**   b.**T**   c.**T**   d.**T**   e.**T**

Nucleoside analogue reverse transcriptase inhibitors are activated by intracellular phosphorylation. Zidovudine/stavudine and lamivudine/zalcitabine are combinations to be avoided since zidovudine interferes with the phosphorylation of stavudine, while lamivudine does the same for zalcitabine.

Ritonavir interferes with the metabolic degradation of many drugs via the cytochrome P450 pathway. It increases the plasma concentration of many substances, including cisapride, terfenadine, amiodarone, flecainide acetate and quinidine. Use of ritonavir with any of these agents is contraindicated. Rifampicin induces this enzyme system and thereby reduces plasma levels of zidovudine.

Blood levels of saquinavir are increased by coadministration with specific brands of single- and double-strength grapefruit juice, which inhibit the intestinal cytochrome P450 enzyme system.

---

137. a.F b.T c.T d.F e.F

Although toxoplasmosis in advanced pregnancy is unlikely to cause major fetal damage it may lead to late congenital disease, especially retinochoroiditis. Toxoplasmosis may be transmitted by fresh blood transfusion and by organ transplantation. PCR of peripheral blood remains positive for about 3 months after initial toxoplasmosis infection. Illness may be accompanied by atypical lymphocytosis; eosinophilia suggests an alternative diagnosis. Reactivated toxoplasmosis, rather than acute infection, accounts for the great majority of cases of toxoplasma encephalitis or brain abscess in AIDS patients.

---

138. a.T b.F c.T d.F e.T

Corticosteroids, when added to antituberculous chemotherapy, slow down the formation of pericardial effusion in tuberculous pericarditis and reduce the need for repeated pericardiocentesis. Controlled clinical trials have demonstrated their ineffectiveness in the Guillain–Barré syndrome.

Systemic corticosteroids, if used early in the treatment of pyogenic meningitis in children, reduce the incidence of neurological sequelae, particularly of auditory nerve damage. Trials have demonstrated this effect most conclusively in *Haemophilus influenzae* type B infection.

Steroid therapy has only a marginal influence on zoster-associated pain and is not recommended.

Treatment is effective in reducing severe pharyngeal oedema in infectious mononucleosis (IM); corticosteroids may also be helpful in treating IM-associated thrombocytopenia and haemolytic anaemia.

---

139. a.T b.T c.T d.F e.T

HIV infection is associated with sensory or mixed neuropathy and mononeuritis multiplex. HIV-induced peripheral nerve damage must be distinguished from HIV myelopathy, cytomegalovirus radiculopathy and neuropathy and from neurotoxic drug side effects.

There is clinical and serological evidence to link *Campylobacter jejuni* infection with polyneuritis, which is also a well-documented complication of diphtheria. Coxsackie viruses have not been conclusively linked to polyneuritis although some serotypes, such as A7, may cause a mild poliomyelitis-like syndrome.

Mononeuritis multiplex is a well-recognized feature of *Borrelia burgdorferi* infection (Lyme disease).

---

140. a.**F** b.**T** c.**F** d.**T** e.**F**

Protease inhibitor monotherapy produces a 1–2 log decrease in HIV viral load which, however, is not sustained. Combination therapy results in a greater and more prolonged suppression of viral replication.

Rifampicin greatly reduces plasma levels of protease inhibitors by enzyme induction of hepatic cytochrome P450. Protease inhibitors may usefully be combined with both nucleoside and non-nucleoside reverse transcriptase inhibitors. Agents such as ritonavir have been shown to reduce mortality when used as add-on therapy for advanced HIV infection. None of this group of drugs achieves high levels in brain or CSF; efficacy in preventing or treating HIV encephalopathy is therefore uncertain.

---

141. a.**T** b.**T** c.**F** d.**F** e.**T**

Oesophagitis in AIDS is most commonly caused by *Candida albicans* and is usually treated empirically with antifungal agents such as fluconazole. Oesophagoscopy is necessary for non-responders; examination may reveal macroscopic or microscopic evidence of either herpes simplex or cytomegalovirus infection. Symptoms suggesting oesophagitis may also result from extensive oesophageal involvement by Kaposi's sarcoma. *Cryptococcus neoformans* and Epstein–Barr virus are not encountered in this situation.

---

142. a.**T** b.**T** c.**T** d.**F** e.**F**

Conjunctivitis and uveitis may complicate shigella dysentery and may be associated with reactive arthropathy. Individuals with the HLA B27 phenotype are more likely to be affected.

Eye complications, including iritis, are common after ophthalmic herpes zoster, particularly if there is involvement of the skin supplied by the nasociliary nerve.

Uveitis, again often in association with reactive polyarthritis, may accompany or follow meningococcal septicaemia. Loiasis is not associated with involvement of the uveal tract although adult worms may migrate visibly through the conjunctiva.

Enterovirus 70 causes severe haemorrhagic conjunctivitis.

---

143. a.**T** b.**F** c.**T** d.**T** e.**F**

Hyposplenism, caused by a number of conditions including coeliac disease and homozygous sickle cell disease, is an indication for pneumococcal vaccine.

Sickle cell trait is not associated with damage to the spleen.

Severe pneumococcal infection is common in alcohol dependency with or without hepatic cirrhosis and such patients merit immunization. HIV-infected individuals are also at risk from pneumococcal disease; pneumococcal vaccination is currently recommended although it has been shown temporarily to increase HIV viral load. Unfortunately the vaccine does not protect against otitis media or recurrent attacks of pneumococcal sinusitis.

---

144. a.**T** b.**T** c.**T** d.**F** e.**T**

A history of animal bite is not invariable in rabies; a bite may have been forgotten or other routes of salivary infection such as mucous membranes or damaged skin may have been involved.

A diagnosis of rabies may be made by immunofluorescent staining of peripheral nerve endings in a skin biopsy, which is usually obtained from the hairline at the neck.

The risk of spread to intensive care staff is not quantifiable but may be prevented by preexposure immunization.

The incubation period of rabies is shorter in children and in adults bitten on the head and neck, since the virus reaches the brain by travelling centripetally along peripheral nerves. Birds and reptiles do not constitute a rabies hazard for human subjects.

---

145. a.**F** b.**F** c.**T** d.**F** e.**F**

Gonococcal arthropathy is caused by a particular strain (auxotype) of *N. gonorrhoeae*. The organism infrequently causes local disease but is well adapted to bloodstream invasion. It is usually fully sensitive to penicillin. Skin lesions may resemble those found in meningococcal septicaemia but are sparser; they contain immune complexes.

The diagnosis is made on clinical grounds and on the result of culture of blood and mucosal sites; serological tests are unreliable. Joint involvement may be oligoarticular and pyogenic or polyarticular and reactive (sterile).

---

146. a.**T** b.**F** c.**T** d.**F** e.**T**

Parvovirus B19 infects bone marrow progenitor cells and causes depression of erythropoiesis. Infection often produces aplastic crises in patients with chronic haemolytic anaemias such as sickle cell disease; in healthy subjects it may be associated with a transient and asymptomatic fall in haemoglobin.

Infection in pregnancy may lead to intrauterine anaemia and hydrops fetalis.

Erythema subitum (roseola infantum) is a benign viral exanthem of young children caused by human herpes virus type 6.

JC virus (a papovavirus) is responsible for one form of chronic encephalopathy in AIDS; the main impact is on cerebral white matter (progressive multifocal leucoencephalopathy).

Persistent parvovirus B19 viraemia has been well documented in a variety of infected individuals; it is associated with prolonged symptoms such as fatigue and arthralgia.

---

147. a.**F** b.**F** c.**T** d.**F** e.**T**

Thrombocytopenia, probably immune mediated, occurs in about 50% of patients with Weil's disease who have renal impairment. Penicillin or tetracycline (doxycycline) therapy may improve renal function in leptospirosis but has not been shown to prevent the need for dialysis in *Leptospira icterohaemor- rhagiae* infection. Bacteraemia is early and transient and blood cultures are usually sterile by the time the patient reaches medical attention. Liver damage is rarely severe; renal impairment is a much more critical factor in clinical management. Myalgic pain is a common feature of Weil's disease and is associated with elevated blood levels of muscle enzymes.

---

148. a.**T** b.**T** c.**F** d.**T** e.**F**

Disseminated or miliary tuberculosis can cause bilateral adrenalitis and adrenal impairment; an adrenocortical crisis may be precipitated by treatment with rifampicin which induces hepatic metabolism of endogenous hydrocortisone. Adrenalitis may also be a feature of cytomegalovirus infection in AIDS and other immunodeficiency states.

Despite the presence of adrenal haemorrhages in meningo-coccal septicaemia (Waterhouse–Friderichsen syndrome) blood levels of adrenocortical hormones are usually elevated.

Five to 10% of patients with subacute progressive histoplas-mosis will develop adrenal insufficiency; patients with AIDS and other causes of immunodeficiency are particularly vulnerable. The staphylococcal toxic shock syndrome is not associated with adrenal failure.

---

149. a.**F** b.**T** c.**T** d.**F** e.**T**

During the first few days of illness, levels of Lassa virus in blood and body fluids are low and the patient does not constitute a major crossinfection hazard. Nevertheless, viraemia can be detected by PCR which often becomes positive by the fourth day. Slow onset and progression is typical of Lassa fever, in contrast with Ebola fever in which onset is abrupt, with haemorrhage occurring relatively early.

If used within the first 7 days of illness, ribavirin (tribavirin) significantly improves survival in Lassa fever compared with historical controls. Fortunately, mortality is lower among secondary cases.

---

150. a.**T** b.**F** c.**F** d.**T** e.**T**

Fluroquinolones are effective against a number of mycobacter-ial species including *Mycobacterium tuberculosis* and the avium-intracellulare complex. Although they are active against food-poisoning salmonellae in vitro, they have little effect on the course of clinical illness. These agents penetrate poorly into CSF and are not used in the treatment of pyogenic meningitis. Achilles tendon rupture is an unusual but well-documented complication of fluoroquinolone usage, particularly in the elderly.

This group of antimicrobials act by inhibiting bacterial DNA gyrase, the enzyme responsible for the final spiral configuration of bacterial nucleic acid.

INDEX

INDEX

Numbers in the index refer to questions not pages. Numbers in italics indicate that specific mention of the subject is made only in the answers section.

A

α1-antitrypsin deficiency, 20
α-feto protein levels, 49
Acalculous cholecystitis, 133
ACE inhibitors, 30, 43
Achilles tendon rupture, 150
Acquired sideroblastic anaemia, *51*
Acromegaly, 44
Activated protein C resistance, 82
Acute intermittent porphyria, 8
Acute-phase reaction, 9
Addison's disease, 26, 29, 30, 32
Adrenal failure, acute, 148
Adrenal hyperplasia, late onset
    congenital, 36
Aedes mosquitoes, 119
African trypanosomiasis, *119*
AIDS, *148*
    acalculous cholecystitis, 133
    encephalopathy, *140*, 146
    indication for VZIG, 129
    microsporidial infection, *111*
    Mycobacterium avium infection, 150
    oesophagitis, 141
    primary intracranial lymphoma, *133*
    progressive multifocal
        leucoencephalopathy, *133*
Albumin, serum concentration, 48
Alcohol, effects on metabolism, 4
Alcoholic liver disease, 9
    cirrhosis, 143
    hepatitis, *49*
Alcoholism, 2, *6*, *53*
Alopecia, 19
Aluminium toxicity, 7, 59
Amoebic liver abscess, 104
Amyloidosis affecting spleen, 83
Anaemia
    aplastic, 51, 84, *85*
    cold-type autoimmune, 61
    haemolytic, 10, *71*, 89, *132*

hypochromic microcytic, 91
iron deficiency, *53*
megaloblastic, 53
microangiopathic haemolytic, 64
microcytic, 79
non-immune acquired haemolytic, 63
pernicious, 25, 52
sideroblastic, 51
warm autoimmune haemolytic, 62
Anatomical blind loop, 52
Androgen excess, *36*
Androgenic alopecia, 19
Angina, 50
Anorexia, 2
Antilymphocyte globulin, side effects
    associated, 85
Antithrombin III deficiency, 98, 99
Aplastic anaemia, 51, 84, *85*
Aplastic crisis, 70
Arboviruses, *114*
ARDS, 85
Arterial blood gas results, 21
Arterial thrombosis, 99, 100
Arteriovenous fistula thrombosis, 60
Ascaris lumbricoides, 124
Ascites, 49
Asthma, indication for VZIG, 129
Atrophic gastritis, 57
Autoimmune haemolytic anaemia, 61, 62
Autoimmune thyroid disease, 107
Autosplenectomy, *73*, *74*, *83*

B

Bacterial infections, iron deficiency, 57
Basophilic stippling, 53
Benzylpenicillin, 126
Bilirubin concentrations, 38
Biochemical tests, interpretation of
    routine, 1
Blackfan-Diamond syndrome, 86
Blackwater fever, *63*
Blood loss, 59
Bone marrow hypoplasia, conditions
    associated, 86
Borrelia burgdorferi, 119, 139
Borrelia duttoni, *119*